Spirituality, Mental Health, and Social Support

Studies in Spiritual Care

Edited by
Simon Peng-Keller, Eckhard Frick,
Christina Puchalski, and John Swinton

Volume 7

Spirituality, Mental Health, and Social Support

A Community Approach

Edited by
Beate Jakob and Birgit Weyel

DE GRUYTER

ISBN 978-3-11-067316-6
e-ISBN (PDF) 978-3-11-067421-7
e-ISBN (EPUB) 978-3-11-067428-6
ISSN 2511-8838

Library of Congress Control Number: 2020940694

Bibliographic information published by the Deutsche Nationalbibliothek
The Deutsche Nationalbibliothek lists this publication in the Deutsche Nationalbibliografie; detailed bibliographic data are available in the Internet at http://dnb.dnb.de.

Typesetting: Integra Software Services Pvt. Ltd.
Printing and binding: CPI books GmbH, Leck

www.degruyter.com

Foreword

This book is the result of many years of cooperation between the *German Institute for Medical Mission* (DIFÄM) in Tübingen, Germany, and the Department of Practical Theology III of the Faculty of Protestant Theology, University of Tübingen. The cooperation included studies on how congregations can identify resources which can promote health with a focus on accompanying people with depression as well as how congregations can be sensitized to mental health and the needs of persons living with mental disorders. In the collaboration, a close connection between research-studies on the one hand and a congregation-based implementation on the other hand was practiced. In this book, we want to share these results of research and experiences with a more international audience, and put them into a wider, complementary context. We are aware that we cannot consider the whole wealth of related inputs coming from English-speaking sources and we cannot cover the whole discussion, but we would like to make a contribution to the discussion from our particular perspective.

The *German Institute for Medical Mission* (DIFÄM)[1] is engaged in health projects in economically poor countries and in neglected areas. For the work in this field it is of great importance to work in a close and continuous cooperation with local partners. Church congregations and local communities are appreciated for the assets they already have and it is the goal to include the strengths of people in local settings and to link communities to the formal health system. The churches are encouraged to recognize their specific contributions and tasks in the field of health and to implement their healing ministry in various contexts today.

From this point of view, the collaboration aimed at the intersections of health and religion, medicine and congregation. The vantage point of the collaboration between DIFÄM and Chair of Practical Theology III has been to focus on the healing ministry of church congregations and local communities, which does not only make sense in neglected areas of the world but also on the doorstep of the Evangelical Church in Germany, that is, closer to Tübingen, in the Evangelical-Lutheran Church in Württemberg. In light of the differentiation of Church and Religion on the one hand as well as the high-level medical system – especially in a university town like Tübingen – on the other hand, it makes sense in our opinion to link both factors. Because of the complexity of structures, functional differentiation is necessary, but the basic approach of our collaboration was to bring both topics into discussion as they stand in relation to each other.

1 For more information: https://difaem.de/1/home/ (last accessed on 1 April 2020).

https://doi.org/10.1515/9783110674217-202

2010–2012 a pilot-project was implemented in Tübingen. This project, in cooperation with Prof. Dr. Gerhard Eschweiler from the Psychiatic clinic and Geriatric Center of the University Tübingen and Dr. Bertold Müller, medical director at the Center for Psychiatry Südwürttemberg, Zwiefalten, had a special focus on depression as an example of mental illness. The purpose was to create a documentation of health resources in church congregations and the promotion of health by congregations using the example of depression. Semi-structured interviews with various groups of people affected by depression, their relatives, volunteers working for institutions caring for people with depression, and volunteers in general were conducted. An online-questionnaire took a closer look at the pastors. Activities in congregations were hosted, workshops for the public were organized, and the results of the survey were evaluated. The experiences and the results of the project were published in 2014.[2]

In 2014 we were given the chance to start the follow-up project "Innovative ways of pastoral care with people with depression" (2014–2015), funded by the Stiftung Diakonie Württemberg. This project was selected as a pilot project for pastoral care (Modellprojekt Seelsorge) by the Evangelical Church in Germany (EKD).[3] As part of this project, we conducted two group-interviews in congregations, and we developed a questionnaire for a quantitative-comparative survey in congregations in Germany as well as in Malawi. We compiled the results of these several surveys in part II (studies).

In the first section of this book, 'Religion and Health. An overview' we present papers from a workshop held in October 2016 in Tübingen which includes Michael Klessmann's lecture on the interrelationship between faith and health from the viewpoint of pastoral care in Practical Theology, and Christian Zwingmann's account of the current state of research in religious psychology. His paper is published in co-authorship with Constantin Klein. Thirdly, Annette Haußmann, who was the project's research assistant, gives insights into the current state of research on spirituality and depression.

As already mentioned, the results of the various surveys are presented in part II. In II.2 (Depression and Pastoral Care from the Viewpoint of Pastors in Germany) we concentrate on and discuss the conclusions of the qualitative interview-study and the results of the online-survey. The results show that pastors are

---

2 Published as a handbook for congregations: Beate Jakob and Birgit Weyel, eds., *Menschen mit Depression. Orientierungen und Impulse für die Praxis in Kirchengemeinden* (Gütersloh: Gütersloher Verlagshaus, 2014). The project was funded by the Lechler Stiftung and the Evangelical-Lutheran Church in Württemberg.

3 The project was also the subject of research. Kerstin Lammer, *Wie Seelsorge wirkt* (Stuttgart: Kohlhammer: 2020).

contact persons for pastoral care and they are faced with mental disorders in diverse situations, including their professional everyday life at their workplace. However, pastoral care is not only limited to the pastors. Realizing the idea of the priesthood of all believers, volunteers also provide spiritual care. Selected insights from one single interview and one group-interview – presented in the form of two case-studies – are given in II.2 (What Motivates Volunteers in Congregations to Take Care of People with Mental Disorder?). Chapter II focuses on people living with mental disorders and their relatives. This contribution presents results from the individual interviews and points out the special experiences and needs of these people.

A quantitative questionnaire allows for a comparative study concerning Malawi and Germany, two totally different cultural contexts with different medical systems (II.4). The focus on Malawi, where DIFÄM is engaged in health care projects, is also part of the research work of Paul Mekani and Japhet Mbaya who present insights into the knowledge about mental disorder and attitudes towards people with mental disorders among health professionals.

The third section of the book addresses the approaches to improve mental health. In addition to providing new insights and findings, the projects have also been engaged in shifting and shaping church congregations and local communities. An opening chapter gives an overview on mental health in a global perspective (III.1). Beate Jakob introduces the developments in three German congregations resulting from events providing information on and raising awareness for mental disorders including special Sunday services, Bible study-groups and other activities of the local church community (III.2). Vandana Kanth's contribution also covers the promotion of mental health on a local level (III.3). Her focus are the communities in the catchment area of the Duncan Hospital in Raxaul (Bihar/India). The studies from Malawi and India are of interest as such. However, they also serve for comparison and correspond to a comparative approach.

The editors are very much indebted to the contributors of this book and the research assistants in the two projects, especially Stefanie Koch and Dr. Annette Haußmann, as well as the student research assistants at the department of Practical Theology and the interns at DIFÄM. Dr. Andreas Kögel (Bayreuth) served as consultant for the quantitative research. We are also especially grateful for the thorough work of Marianne Schweitzer-Martin and her careful attention revising the texts.

Many people in church congregations and local communities supported our work: Professor Dr. Gerhard Eschweiler (psychiatrist) and Professor Dr. Martin Hautzinger (psychologist) from the University of Tübingen provided valuable advice over recent years, as well as the hospital chaplain Friedemann

Bresch (Tübingen) who was an advisor to the project. The pastors, volunteers and especially the people affected by mental disorders supported us with a great openness.

We received generous funding for our work from the Lechler Stiftung, Stiftung Diakonie Württemberg and the Evangelical-Lutheran Church in Württemberg. We express our sincere gratitude to all who made this work possible.

Last but not least, we thank the editors of this series for admission and the publishing house De Gruyter.

Beate Jakob (DIFÄM) and Birgit Weyel
(Practical Theology at the Faculty of
Protestant Theology, Eberhard Karls
University, Tübingen)

Contents

Beate Jakob and Birgit Weyel

Introduction

Spirituality, Mental Health, and Social Support. A Community Approach

The relation between religion and (mental) health as a subject of science is multiplex und multi-layered. It has been dealt with in religious psychology, philosophy, medicine and theology for a long time; in the German-speaking context it had a fruitful, interdisciplinary origin and a further development marked by a breaking off and discontinuity in the 20th century.[1] Since the 1990s, a growing interest in empirical research on the relation between religion and mental health has been observed,[2] but there are some problems which inhibit research to a great extent: e.g. the conceptualization of religiosity[3] with its manifold social and psychological dimensions.[4] While religious psychology in the USA is a very lively field of research, the cultural background and the basic conditions of religious practice are very different, so that the religious studies performed in the USA cannot simply be transferred to our German context. Christian Zwingmann and Constantin Klein give insights into the connection betweenreligion and health from the perspective of psychology of religion with regard to the cultural context.[5]

---

1 Cf. Christian Henning, "Die Geschichte der Religionspsychologie im deutschsprachigen Raum," in *Einführung in die Religionspsychologie*, eds. Christian Henning, Sebastian Murken and Erich Nestler (Paderborn: Schöningh, 2003): 9–90.

2 Cf. Marion Schowalter and Sebastian Murken, "Religion und psychische Gesundheit," in *Einführung in die Religionspsychologie*, eds. Christian Henning, Sebastian Murken and Erich Nestler (Paderborn: Schöningh, 2003): 138–162, 141.

3 Cf. Schowalter and Murken, "Religion und psychische Gesundheit," 143 and Franz Buggle, "Warum gibt es (fast) keine deutsche empirische Religionspsychologie," *Forschungsberichte des Psychologischen Instituts der Albert-Ludwigs-Universität Freiburg i. Br. 73* (1991).

4 Stefan Huber has developed a reliable model for research, which integrates social and psychic dimensions of religiosity (model of centrality); cf. Stefan Huber, *Dimensionen der Religiosität: Skalen, Messmodelle und Ergebnisse einer empirisch orientierten Religionspsychologie* (Bern/Göttingen: Huber, 1996). Cf. also Stefan Huber and Constantin Klein, "Spirituelle und religiöse Konstrukträume," in *Spiritualität transdisziplinär. Wissenschaftliche Grundlagen im Zusammenhang mit Gesundheit und Krankheit*, eds. Arndt Büssing and Niko Kohls (Berlin/Heidelberg: Springer-Verlag, 2011): 53–66. Cf. the overview Constantin Klein, Sonja Gottschling and Christian Zwingmann, "Deutschsprachige Fragebögen zur Messung von Religiosität/Spiritualität. Ein empirisch gestützter Vergleich ausgewählter Skalen," *Spiritual Care* 1.3 (2012): 22–35. Cf. also Mirjam Hoffmann, *Religiosität und psychische Gesundheit* (Stuttgart: Kohlhammer, 2019).

5 Cf. Chapter I.2 in this volume: Christian Zwingmann and Constantin Klein, *Religion and Health from the View of Psychology of Religion: Empirical Results – Possible Pathways – Cultural Context.*

https://doi.org/10.1515/9783110674217-001

Nevertheless, in the last decades some studies on the relationship between religion and mental health have been carried out in the German-speaking context as well.[6] Furthermore, under the designation of *Spiritual Care* a remarkable number of studies were published over the last years. Particularly with regard to hospital pastoral care, a strong cooperation between spiritual care given by multiprofessional teams and academic surveys on spirituality can be observed. The SPIR-questionnaire, for example, is a method, which addresses counselling as well as research knowledge with regard to the spiritual needs and resources of patients in health facilities. SPIR – an acronym – consists of a semi-structured interview that focuses on the religious or rather spiritual beliefs (Spirituality), how important these beliefs are for the life of a person, the affiliation to a religious community and the perception of the role of doctors and pastors.[7]

This concept of spiritual care favours an idea of spirituality, which is less focussed on individual religiosity and understands religion in multiple ways in light of multicultural contexts. Traugott Roser points out: "Spirituality is first of all perceived as a difference: as a distinguishing feature among people who would call themselves spiritual but have a very different understanding of the term, not least independent from their religious socialisation and biography."[8]

---

6 Cf. Annette Dörr, "Religiosität und psychische Gesundheit. Zur Zusammenhangsstruktur spezifischer religiöser Konzepte," *Studienreihe psychologische Forschungsergebnisse Band 80* (Hamburg: Verlag Dr. Kovac, 2001); and Sebastian Murken, *Gottesbeziehung und psychische Gesundheit. Die Entwicklung eines Modelles und seine empirische Überprüfung* (Münster/ New York: Waxmann, 1998).

7 Cf. Traugott Roser, *Spiritual Care. Der Beitrag von Seelsorge zum Gesundheitswesen* (Stuttgart: Kohlhammer, [2]2017), 391–398. It must be pointed out that the questionaire has been developed in the context of palliative care but it can be taken as an example for a multi-professional approach. SPIR refers to FICA, a guideline, developed by Christina Puchalski's team. FICA represents the main components of the questionnaire: faith and belief, importance, community und adress/action in care. See Christina Puchalski and Anna Romer, "Taking a spiritual history allows clinicians to understand patients more fully," *Journal of Palliative Medicine* 3 (2000): 129–137. See also Christina Puchalski, "Spiritual Care: Practical tools," in *A time for listening and caring: Spirituality and the care of the chronically ill and dying*, ed. Christina Puchalski (Oxford/New York: Oxford University Press, 2006): 229–251. Cf. also René Hefti, "Spiritualität und Medizin. Ein empirischer Beitrag zur Spiritualitätsforschung," in *Spiritualität im Diskurs. Spiritualitätsforschung in theologischer Perspektive*, eds. Ralph Kunz and Claudia Kohli Reichenbach (Zürich: Theologischer Verlag Zürich, 2012): 241–261.

8 "Spiritualität wird dabei zunächst als Differenz erfahrbar: Als Unterscheidungsmerkmal zwischen Menschen, die sich zwar als spirituell bezeichnen, den Begriff jedoch ganz unterschiedlich füllen, unabhängig nicht zuletzt von ihrer religiösen Sozialisation und ihrer Biographie"; Roser, *Spiritual Care*, 399 (trans. Birgit Weyel).

Spirituality is therefore, first of all, experienced as difference: as the differentiating characteristic between humans, who indeed identify themselves as spiritual, however fill the term in very different ways, independently – not only – of their religious socialization and their biography.

The blending of the terms spirituality and spiritual care is helpful when focusing on the individual's beliefs and needs in a multi-professional context, whereas a strict boundary between pastoral care and spiritual care does not make sense.[9] The contribution of Michael Klessmann from the perspective of practical theology's poimenics on the relation between faith and healing shows that pastoral care is already concerned with the overlap of the relevant issues in the field of pastoral care and chaplaincy for sick people.[10] Health as well is not only a medical issue, but has various connections with religion and spirituality, as we would like to show. The approach in this book is to show intersections particularly with regard to religion and spirituality and health, as well as health-care and communities. Below we will introduce this approach to health and community.

Specialization in modern societies is connected with a required differentiation between religion (church) and health (medicine). We do not want to put this into question but would like to show that there is not only a relation between health and spirituality with regard to content, but also that congregations provide support for (mental) health and vice versa: medical facilities can also benefit from a stronger cooperation with congregations. Congregations are complex social entities with connecting factors to medicine, welfare and social work and pastoral care. There might be differences in the health care delivery system for examples in Germany and Malawi,[11] but a community approach to health makes sense here and there. Congregations – so the basic assumption – can contribute to health through providing health-related information and for social as well as spiritual reasons. The concern of this book is the indication of a congregational approach regarding mental health as a helpful addition to other

---

9 It does not make sense to play pastoral care off against spiritual care and vice versa. Cf. Doris Nauer, *Spiritual Care statt Seelsorge?* (Stuttgart: Kohlhammer, 2015). Cf. also the differentiated statement of Eberhardt Hauschildt regarding similarities and differences: Eberhard Hauschildt, "'Spiritual Care' – eine Herausforderung für die Seelsorge?" *Materialdienst der EZW* 3 (2013): 83–90.

10 Cf. chapter I.1 in this volume: Michael Klessmann, *Does Faith Heal? Reflections on the Complex Relationship of Religion, Illness and Health.*

11 Cf. chapter II.4 in this volume: Annette Haußmann, Beate Jakob, and Birgit Weyel, *Spirituality, Congregational Support and Mental Health – the Example of Depression. Results of a Comparative Study among Volunteers in Congregations and Professionals in Healthcare Settings, Conducted in Germany and Malawi.*

academic initiatives "to promote general awareness among researchers, scholars and professionals of the importance of religious and spiritual issues."[12]

That health is not only a medical issue, has not only been promoted by theology and sociology, but by medicine itself. This position is stated in the definition of health developed by the World Health Organization (WHO).

1 The Definition of Health by the WHO

What is health? Which factors impact health positively or negatively? How can the health status of individuals and of the society be improved? In the middle of the 20th century when the world faced a striking disparity in global health, the World Health Organization (WHO) and the churches put these questions on their agenda. Up to the middle of the 20th century, health had been almost exclusively the domain of scientific medicine and health professionals. Health work was shaped by a static concept of health saying that, "Health is the absence of disease." According to such a narrow understanding of health, healing was mainly restricted to curing diseases. This understanding of health and the corresponding one-dimensional approach to health however was questioned when it became obvious that a curative and institutional-based approach to health alone had not improved global health but instead had led to a striking discrepancy between the health status of people in the industrialized countries and those living in resource-limited countries or regions.

In the constitution of the WHO health was defined as "a complete state of physical, mental, and social well-being and not merely the absence of disease or infirmity."[13] At the same time, the WHO called for access to health for all by stating, "the enjoyment of the highest attainable standard of health – is one of the fundamental rights of every human being."

The WHO definition of health has often been blamed as being utopian. However, this critique is not aware of the definition's true intention: Such a broad view challenges a purely curative approach to health and calls for a multi-dimensional approach. Health is not only a medical issue. This means that in their efforts to improve health in a sustainable way, the governments

12 E.g.: René Hefti and Arndt Büssing, eds., "Integrating Religion and Spirituality into Clinical Practice. Conference Proceedings. European Conference on Religion, Spirituality and Health," in URL: https://doi.org/10.3390/books978-3-03842-929-6 (last accessed on 1 April 2020).

13 WHO, *Preamble to the Constitution of WHO as adopted by the International Health Conference* (New York, 19 June – 22 July 1946).

should apply a comprehensive approach. The medical work offered by hospitals and other health institutions needs to be complemented by considering and addressing the factors contributing positively or negatively to health. These include sanitation, nutrition, safe water and also education and poverty reduction.

But instead of the WHO definition of health influencing health policies of governments, the decades after World War II were shaped by an adverse development. Especially in the industrialized countries, health systems were still marked by an over-reliance on costly medical technology and an over-estimation of the curative approach to health. As a consequence of this prevailing "Western model" of health care, the world faced an ever growing disparity in terms of access to health services and health status between countries and also within countries.

The unjust global health situation also alarmed the churches and the representatives of Christian health care. During the 1960s and 1970s, the World Council of Churches (WCC) in cooperation with the German Institute for Medical Mission (DIFÄM) called for conferences to address this situation and develop new concepts of Christian Health Care. In 1968, the WCC established the Christian Medical Commission (CMC) as its health desk. In their search for alternative concepts for addressing health disparities and improving global health during the 1960s and 1970s, the WHO effectively cooperated with representatives of the CMC. They formed a think tank that developed the concept of Primary Health Care (PHC) presented at the World Health Assembly in Alma Ata in 1978.

With the vision of "Health for All by the Year 2000", the Alma Ata Declaration articulated PHC as a set of principles for the reformation of health services and for addressing priority health needs and the fundamental determinants of health.[14] The Alma Ata Declaration is based on a set of values – equity, social justice, universal access and solidarity – and reveals the following important principles of a comprehensive approach to public health:

- Inter-sectoral approach: With regard to any attempt to improve health, it is recommended to take the determinants of health like sanitation, nutrition, water, education and economic factors into account.
- Participation: PHC is people-centered. Instead of offering interventions in a top-down manner, PHC is a bottom-up approach to health whereby people at the local level are the main actors. It gives space for solutions created and owned by communities which use their own strengths. Individuals and communities have both a right and an obligation to take part in decisions and actions that affect their health.

14 Cf. WHO, *Primary Health Care. Report of the International Conference on Primary Health Care, Alma Ata, USSR, 6–12 September* (Geneva: World Health Organization, 1978).

– Health care is most effective if it integrates health promotion as well as preventive and curative interventions.

In 1986, the WHO Ottawa Charter on Health Promotion[15] resumed the principles of the Alma Ata Declaration and developed the concept of health promotion further. This charter defines health promotion as the "process of enabling people to increase control over, and to improve their health."

Disease prevention addresses the risk factors to health like unhealthy living conditions, drug and alcohol abuse, bacterial and viral infection agents, etc. Health promotion stands for a concept that focusses on strengthening those social and individual factors that have the potential to improve health like conducive work place conditions, physical exercise, healthy diets, life skills, etc. There are of course overlaps between disease prevention and health promotion so that it is not possible to differentiate precisely between the two. However, while preventive measures are mainly to be planned and implemented by the medical system, health promotion is not just the responsibility of the health sector but "is shared among individuals, community groups, health professionals, health service institutions and governments." Moreover, the Ottawa Charter states that, "health is created and lived by people within the settings of their everyday life." Thus, the concept of health promotion clearly counts on individuals and communities to be active partners of the medical system towards improving health of individuals and societies.

Health promotion is a resource-oriented instead of a deficit-oriented approach to health. It corresponds with the concepts of salutogenesis and resilience that today are widely applied in psychology, pedagogy and other social sciences.[16]

The Alma Ata Declaration as well as the Ottawa Charter marked a breakthrough in public health as they broadened the medical model to include social and economic factors and as it put health equity on the international political agenda. In the 1980s, many people and organizations that were active in global health showed great appreciation of this new approach and believed it had the potential to effectively address the global health inequities.

15 WHO, *The Ottawa Charter for Health Promotion. First International Conference on Health Promotion* (Ottawa, 21 November 1986); in URL: http://www.who.int/healthpromotion/conferences/previous/ottawa/en/ (last accessed on 1 April 2020).

16 Cf. e.g. Friedrich Riffer, Elmar Kaiser, Manuel Sprung and Lore Streibl, eds., *Das Fremde: Flucht – Trauma – Resilienz. Aktuelle traumaspezifische Konzepte in der Psychosomatik. Psychosomatik im Zentrum* (Berlin/Heidelberg: Springer, 2018).

However, the concept of PHC was misunderstood from the beginning. It was regarded as an attack on the medical establishment and was confused with an exclusive focus on first-level care. Some people regarded PHC as utopian, and many in the industrialized countries thought PHC was cheap and poor care for poor people – a "second class" health care for people in developing countries while the countries in the Global North were priviledged to enjoy high standard health services offered by well-functioning mostly curative medical services. But, also most governments in low-income countries continued to concentrate their efforts on building up medical institutions offering curative health services. In the 1980s and 1990s, still an optimistic view of the medical approach prevailed all over the world. Development work in the medical field aimed at making high-standard medicine available also in resource-limited settings. It was assumed that scientific medicine would develop even further to finally be able to cure most of the diseases all over the world.

40 years after the declaration of Alma Ata, the WHO reaffirmed its commitment to PHC in the Global Conference on Primary Health Care held in Astana, October 2018. The Declaration of Astana recommends the implementation of PHC as an important contribution to reaching "Health for All". It says: "We are convinced that strengthening primary health care (PHC) is the most inclusive, effective and efficient approach to enhance people's physical and mental health, as well as social well-being, and that PHC is a cornerstone of a sustainable health system for universal health coverage (UHC) and health-related Sustainable Development Goals."[17]

2 A Christian Definition of Health

During the 1970s and 1980s, the CMC convened worldwide discussions on the Christian understanding of health, healing and healing community. These discussions reflected the spirit of Alma Ata and brought out a concept of a healing community and congregation which is also of relevance today.

The ecumenical discussions were summarized in the document "Healing and Wholeness. The Churches' Role in Health" which was adopted by the WCC and published in 1989. In this publication, health is defined as "a dynamic state of wellbeing of the individual and the society; of physical, mental,

17 URL: https://www.who.int/docs/default-source/primary-health/declaration/gcphc-declaration.pdf (last accessed on 1 April 2020).

spiritual, economic, political and social well-being; of being in harmony with each other, with the material environment, and with God."[18]

This comprehensive definition of health builds on the WHO definition, but adds some new elements. Health is no longer seen as an individual affair, but the well-being of the individual is seen in direct relation to the way society is constituted. Moreover and very importantly, the CMC definition of health includes the spiritual dimension of health.

Furthermore, this definition assumes that health is not a static concept by which we can distinguish clearly between those who are healthy and those who are not; rather, every person is in constant flux between various levels of maintaining health and fighting infection and disease, hence the term "dynamic state". This kind of process-oriented understanding of health reflects the concept of health promotion.

This Christian understanding of health has consequences for the understanding of the church's mission: It means that, alongside the practices of scientific and also the so-called alternative medicine, churches and congregations have both resources and tasks in the field of health and healing. The document states that "most churches today preach and teach but have abdicated healing to medical professionals. Yet [there are] many ways in which churches are involved in healing."[19]

Faith communities can contribute to health in various ways:
- Congregations are social networks with the potential to turn in solidarity towards sick, lonely, handicapped, oppressed, and marginalized and to those with social problems such as divorce, unemployment, unplanned pregnancy, etc.
- Congregations are places where people come together to worship, to pray for each other, to share about faith, and to commonly search for the meaning of life.
- The congregation is a teaching place by, e.g., facilitation self-discovery of causes of ill health; practical health education; studying questions of biomedical ethics; learning to take personal responsibility for health.[20]

The document advocates for "health in the hands of the people" and explicitly refers to Primary Health Care by stating that "congregations are urged to be involved in and promote primary health care (PHC) as a means of correcting the

18 WCC (World Council of Churches), *Healing and Wholeness – The Churches Role in Health. The Report of a Study by the Christian Medical Commission* (Geneva: WCC, 1990), 6.
19 WCC, *Healing and Wholeness*, 30–31.
20 Cf. WCC, *Healing and Wholeness*, 30–31.

existing unjust distribution of health care resources. Through PHC, persons in all places in the world can be empowered to discover the causes of most of their illness and eliminate them. Through PHC the heavy dependence on professional and institutional health services can be lifted, allowing them to provide more expert care for the complicated illnesses for which they are trained and equipped."[21]

The concept of PHC has offered a huge chance to the churches as they have the infrastructure to implement PHC through their congregations and – as pointed out above – contribute to health through spiritual and social support and provide valuable health information. Thus, churches can be vital partners of the government health system. However, like the governments, up to now the churches all over the world have not been ready to engage in the implementation of PHC on a large scale. Moreover, many churches are no longer very clear about their role in health and sometimes they even consider handing over their health facilities and thus their healing ministry to government health services.

3 The Discussion of the Spiritual Dimension of Health within the WHO

The CMC definition of health approved in 1989 explicitly includes the spiritual dimension of health while the 1946 WHO definition does not mention it. Up to now, the WHO has not amended its definition though there have been repeated inquiries about it. These inquiries reflected the fact that in most cultures health has a spiritual dimension and has always been included in health services.

During the WHO General Assembly in 1983, the participants intensively discussed the extension of the WHO definition of health by including the spiritual dimension. That a WHO assembly put issues of spirituality, which so far had been excluded from the public health discourse, on its agenda was due to the influence of the then WHO General Secretary Dr Halfdan Mahler who was very much open for including the spiritual dimension in the definition of health as well as in health programs. Due to Mahler's efforts, in 1984 the WHO approved a resolution (WHA 37.13) that recommended its member states to include the spiritual dimension in their strategies towards improving health and reaching the goal of "Health for All". Though this resolution was not more than a recommendation, it marked a milestone in the WHO history as it broadens the so far predominantly scientific approach to health by an

---

21 WCC, *Healing and Wholeness*, 32–33.

immaterial dimension that is not easy to measure and sometimes even difficult to understand and describe.

Only 14 years later, in 1998, the WHO discussed the question of amending the WHO health definition given in the preamble of the WHO Constitution by including the spiritual dimension. A WHO working group drafted resolution EB 101.R2 that suggested the following new definition of health to become part of the Constitution: "Health is a dynamic state of complete physical, mental, spiritual and social well-being and not merely the absence of disease and infirmity."[22] The influence of the CMC definition on this suggested definition of health is obvious in that it mentions the spiritual dimension and regards health as a dynamic state.

Resolution EB 192.R2 again appeared on the agenda of the WHO 52. General Assembly and was discussed intensively. While most representatives of the member states in the Global South strongly supported the definition, some of those speaking for the states in the North, for example the Soviet Union, were hesitant to include the spiritual dimension in the official WHO health definition. They regarded spirituality to belong to one's private sphere instead of being taken into account in the public health discourse. As a result, there was no majority for the amendment of the health definition in the WHO Constitution. Instead, the responsible committee suggested keeping this question on the WHO agenda.

In the years to follow, the question repeatedly came up again, for example in a round table discussion during the 58. WHO Assembly in 2005 (The Round Table Spirituality, Religion and Health 2005). Moreover, in his opening address to the 61. Assembly in 2008, Archbishop Desmond Tutu (South Africa) encouraged the WHO to finally add the spiritual dimension to its health definition. However, up to now the 1946 definition of health has remained the official WHO health definition.[23]

---

22 WHO, "Review of the Constitution and Regional Arrangements of the World Health Organization Executive Board 101st Session," EB 101/7 (Geneva: 1997).

23 To the WHO discussions cf. Beate Jakob and Peter Bartmann, "Gesundheit und Gesundheitsförderung. Ansätze zu einer Integration der spirituellen Dimension in Konzepte und die Arbeit der WHO," in *Spiritualität und seelische Gesundheit*, eds. J. Armbruster et al. (Köln: Psychiatrie Verlag, 2013): 48–62; Simon Peng-Keller, "Spiritual Care im Gesundheitswesen des 20. Jahrhunderts. Von der sozialen Medizin zur WHO-Diskussion um die 'spirituelle Dimension'," in *Spiritual Care im globalisierten Gesundheitswesen. Historische Hintergründe und aktuelle Entwicklungen*, eds. S. Peng-Keller and D. Neuhold (Darmstadt: Wissenschaftliche Buchgesellschaft, 2019): 13–72.

4 Today's Health Situation and the Concept of Religious Health Assets

Until today, the medical system has not met the great expectations put to it. In the countries of the Global South many people still lack access to quality health services and essential medicines. The progress that was made in medicine benefitted not all countries and regions equally. Instead, the disparities between and in countries are still there.

But also in the industrialized countries, the health situation and the way health systems work are far from being perfect. For example, chronic diseases including mental disorders are on the rise and many people have to live and cope with them. With regard to chronic diseases, the patient's family also (to varying degrees) take on a share of the responsibility. Society must react to these altered patterns in the progress of disease and has to search for ways to include the sick and the disabled in society and in professional life and to provide care and help beyond cure.

The exorbitant costs of the medical system in the North are another problem that has created a huge challenge for the society. Therefore, the WHO and other global health organizations still strongly emphasize the need to move from a purely curative approach to health to prevention and health promotion.

This situation provides a new window of opportunity to globally think about new approaches to health by including the contribution of communities and congregations. This is an opportunity but also a challenge as we can only encourage congregations to promote health if they know exactly how they can do so.

Churches and Christian communities significantly contribute to health, especially in resource-limited settings. However, Christian health services are not always aligned with the formal health system. While most governments appreciate Christian health services, only a few are ready to allocate an appropriate share of the national health budget to the health work of the churches.

These are just some of the reasons:

- Historically, the churches themselves did not actively seek a close cooperation with the formal health system, especially as long as they had enough funds from other, mostly overseas sources.
- So far, the churches' contribution to health has not been documented properly. Most of their huge health work, especially the work of communities, is literally not "on the map."
- Sometimes, there has also been a problem of communication between governments and the churches. Representatives of the governments might say

that, "these church people are people of good will who do a lot of good. We need them. But nobody knows exactly what they are doing. It's sometimes even difficult to understand them as they use their own faith language."

- Moreover, faith communities themselves often are not aware of what they actually contribute to health.

How then can we understand and document the contribution of faith communities to health? How can we make this contribution known to the communities themselves as well as to the public? These questions led to establishing the "African Religious Health Assets Programme" (ARHAP) in 2001; today known as "International Religious Health Assets Programme" (IRHAP).[24] IRHAP is a collaborative research network based at the University of Cape Town. Its aim is to document the contribution of religion and of religious communities to health, and to align church-based health services with the formal health system.

The introduction of the idea of Religious Health Assets (RHAs) is based on the assumption that religions and religious communities have health related resources, potentials, capabilities, strengths that they own like a financial capital (= an asset) to work with. These assets can be active or they can be there without being used. In the latter case, they need to be activated like a financial asset that is at one's disposal and needs to be invested.

According to IRHAP, faith communities contribute to health because they own "Religious Health Assets" (RHAs). In Biblical terms assets are the "talents" of faith communities that can promote health. These assets or talents can be tangible or intangible.

Tangible or visible health assets of faith communities like the provision of medical services or groups caring for others are well known and appreciated. In addition, faith communities own so-called intangible, invisible health assets. These are rooted in the spiritual dimension and the motivational and mobilizing capacity of faith communities. These assets like trust, motivation, credibility, compassion, mutual support, honesty, prayer, moral authority, etc. can play an important part in fostering the health of individuals and communities. However, as it is difficult to assess these assets and to measure their impact on health, they are often overlooked.

24 URL: http://www.irhap.uct.ac.za/ (last accessed on 1 April 2020).

Within the framework of ARHAP's research programme, a matrix was developed to thoroughly examine the issue of religious health assets from the perspective of the African continent. With some minor alterations, this matrix can also be applied to the European context.

In table 1, the tangible and intangible health assets described above are put along the vertical axis. As both tangible and intangible health assets can have a direct or indirect impact on health, the health assets are put in different positions along the horizontal axis. This then produces four quadrants, which show the health assets and their positive outcomes.

Table 1: Religious Health Assets Matrix.*

Intangible Assets	***Intangible assets with a direct impact on health***	***Intangible assets with an indirect impact on health***
	Prayer Time for sick people Health awareness Being prepared to help Sensitivity to problems ...	Personal sense of meaning in life Social contacts Feeling of belonging to God/other people Openness to social or political issues Hope Trust.
Tangible Assets	***Tangible assets with a direct impact on health***	***Tangible assets with an indirect impact on health***
	Hospitals and Health Centres Care, Counselling, etc. Parish centres that are open to all Room for self-help groups Leisure opportunities for disabled people ...	Educational/training opportunities Choir and other fellowships Religious services providing a structure to the week Sacraments and rituals providing structure in times of crisis ...
	Direct impact	***Indirect impact***
	Positive impact on health	

*Adaptation of a matrix developed by Jim Cochrane. Cf. Jim Cochrane, "Religious Health Assets (RHAs) – Conceptual and Theoretical Framework," in *Religion, Faith and Public Health. Documentation on a Consultation held at Difäm*, ed. Difäm, German Institute for Medical Mission (Tübingen, 9–11 February 2006): 14–45, 24.

Talking about the impact on health, one usually refers to the assets in the bottom-left quadrant of the matrix which are the tangible health assets with a direct positive impact on health, e.g. hospitals, care and counselling groups, etc. These assets can be measured and quantified. Among the tangible health assets having an indirect impact on health are, for instance, groups that create relationships, like the choir which can also have a positive impact on health, and rituals. These tangible assets are usually not regarded as health promoting, but they often do have a positive impact on health.

The two upper quadrants refer to intangible religious health assets, graded according to their direct or indirect impact on health – like prayer and resilience, which are directly related to health, and a sense of meaning and faith/hope/love which are assets not directly linked to health, but with a major impact on health. These assets are much more difficult to assess than the tangible ones as they are not quantifiable but have to be assessed through qualitative methods.

The RHA matrix was initially designed to demonstrate and document the contribution of faith communities to health with regard to HIV and AIDS. For people living with HIV and AIDS it is obviously very important to have access to treatment and care. But we also know that belonging to a social network as well as having hope and trust affects these patients' physical and even more their mental health significantly.

Rather than being a classification system, the matrix can serve as an eye-opener that helps to widen the understanding of health promotion by faith communities. Health promotion cannot be narrowed down to, e.g., praying for the sick nor can it be restricted to providing space for self-help groups as an example of a tangible health asset with a direct impact on health. Moreover, this concept demonstrates that the genuine contribution of faith communities to health is not a special task, an add-on to what is being done already. The majority of these religious health assets, especially the intangible ones, are an integral part of everyday life of the community. The community as a social network and a place of worship is a healing place in itself.

Looking at the various and specific ways in which faith communities contribute to health also helps to overcome the understanding of the churches' and faith communities' contribution to health being in competition to medicine and the formal health system. Church health services and the contribution to health provided by congregations reflect a holistic approach to health that adds value to the medical approach and cannot be replaced by it.

5 A Holistic Approach to Mental Health

All over the world, the burden of mental disorders is growing. According to the WHO, depression is the leading cause of disability worldwide and a major contributor to the overall global burden of disease. Worldwide, more than 300 million people are affected.[25]

As an example, the reports of health insurances provide alarming figures: While the total of sick days in Germany has decreased over the past ten years, sick leave due to mental disorders has increased considerably – their share of the total sick leave has gone up from 2 to more than 15 percent.[26] While other diseases report an absence of 12 days on the average, absence due to mental diseases is 36 days on average.[27]

What is true for each disease, is especially true for mental disorders: They are not only a medical issue. Of course, a professional therapy of mental disorders is indispensable. But, at the same time, many health professionals including psychiatrists and psychotherapists point to the fact that a professional therapy can and should be complemented by, for example, social support, values that give a hold in life, sport and music. This insight helps to recognize ways in which congregations in their capacity of being social networks and providing values, and also various forms of church music own religious health assets that can promote mental health in cooperation with health professionals.

6 The Congregations' Contribution to Health

Based on the insight that health is not only a medical issue and the concept of the Religious Health Assets, we can describe the possible contribution to health offered by congregations under two aspects: Congregations are (a) social networks and they are (b) places for interpretation of life and health and related disorders.

6.1 Congregations Are Social Networks

Mental diseases are still very often treated as a taboo. This has consequences whether people make use of medical treatment or not and the way people living with mental disorders and their relatives are perceived. Firstly, congregations are social networks in which people can share and access information about

25 Cf. URL: http://www.who.int/mediacentre/factsheets/fs369/en/ (last accessed on 1 April 2020).
26 Cf. Franz Knieps and Holger Pfaff, *Gesundheit und Arbeit. Zahlen, Daten, Fakten,* BKK Gesundheitsreport 2016 (Berlin: Medizinisch Wissenschaftliche Verlagsgesellschaft, 2016), 59.
27 Cf. Knieps and Pfaff, *Gesundheit und Arbeit*, 47.

mental diseases and gain awareness of the problems mentally sick people must deal with. In congregations there are people with mental problems as well as in the general population. Perhaps the percentage is even higher in congregations because there are low-threshold services, drop-in centres and counselling for people with problems, groups for bereaved, etc. There are many entry points for more information and awareness training. As the studies in Germany as well as in Malawi show, information and knowledge is needed and can help to reduce prejudices and discrimination.

Pastors, volunteers and other staff members, like the secretary in the parish office and the caretaker in the parish hall can work as multipliers in the field of mental disorders and have an influence so that the congregation works like a social network benefitting others through help, support and a friendly inclusiveness for people and their needs.[28]

The attributes mentioned above are not exclusive for church-communities, they can also be significant for other social groups, associations, etc. Beyond that and more specifically, church communities are places of lived religion.[29] Congregations are faith-based communities, Christian communities desire to be church in the world, by celebrating God's gift of salvation, which includes all people and endows a special connectedness and openness for others. Actually this is not implemented everywhere, but it is the main principle of Christian belief which has to be kept in mind.[30] Congregations are open spaces, where meaning and purpose can be discovered, in a sense of the individual and as a common quest. They bear in remembrance a transcendent dimension of life.

---

28 Cf. chapter II.1. in this volume: Annette Hausmann, Beate Jakob, and Birgit Weyel, *Depression and Pastoral Care from the Viewpoint of Pastors in Germany* and chapter II.2. in this volume: Birgit Weyel, *What Motivates Volunteers in Congregations to Take Care of People with Mental Disorders? Looking at Pastoral Counselling Done by Volunteers in Local Congregations.*

29 Cf. for the concept Wilhelm Gräb's study: Wilhelm Gräb, *Lebensgeschichten – Lebensentwürfe – Sinndeutungen. Eine Praktische Theologie gelebter Religion* (Gütersloh: Gütersloher Verlagshaus,[2]2000) and for the South-African context: Daniël Louw, "'Verbing God' within the dynamics of 'Lived Religion'. 'Sympathetic Rites of Passage' in a Practical Theological approach to the complexity of everyday life," in *Pluralisation and social change. Dynamics of lived religion in South Africa and in Germany,* Praktische Theologie im Wissenschaftsdiskurs Bd. 21, eds. Lars Charbonnier, Johan Cilliers, Matthias Mader, Cas Wepener and Birgit Weyel (Berlin: De Gruyter, 2018): 51–65.

30 Louw, "'Verbing God' within the dynamics of 'Lived Religion'," 52: "Faith as a dynamic of lived religion and praxis of divine experiences; religious experiences as an expression of 'piety' and humane self-understanding."

"The experience of connection with something greater than oneself can be a spiritual resource and ignite a resilient response."[31]

In the New Testament, there are terms and propositions which refer to the transcendent community with God in Christ.[32] These verses, as the arguments and quarrels in early Christianity show, do not describe the factual condition of the congregations as empirical formations and human entities, but they can realize community in the sense of a higher order, so to say 'in heaven', which is constituted by God with relevance also for shaping interpersonal relationships and living together. According to the New Testament, the integration into the heavenly community brings people from different social contexts and roles together and unites them: "There is neither Jew nor Greek, there is neither bond nor free, there is neither male nor female: for ye are all one in Christ Jesus" (Gal 3,28).

The spiritual character of Christian communities is not only but in a very special way symbolized through celebrating the sacraments: Baptism means the emblematic incorporation in the body of Christ, Holy Communion is a reminder of the Last Supper of the disciples with Christ and includes the communicants in the heavenly worship, singing together in communion with angels and saints. These are strong symbols for inclusion of people into Christian communities and shaping social life in congregations.[33]

The theological perspective is essential for many reasons. One reason is to make sure that the social and spiritual support of people who are living with (mental) diseases is the very center of Christian life and not another duty and burden they have to shoulder. In times of dealing with fewer church members, less money and staff – as is the case with the churches in Germany -, two things are important: to make sure that this task takes on a realistic dimension of a congregation's life and that there are assets that congregations already have.

In recent times, critical voices have been raised concerning the so-called "charitable view" (diakonischer Blick). In contrast, a strong pleading for a "decharitabilization of the perception of challenged persons"[34] (Entdiakonisierung

---

31 Yolanda Dreyer, "Material poverty and the poverty of excess: Meaning-making as healing in an era of supermodernism," in *Pluralisation and social change. Dynamics of lived religion in South Africa and in Germany*, Praktische Theologie im Wissenschaftsdiskurs Bd. 21, eds. Lars Charbonnier, Johan Cilliers, Matthias Mader, Cas Wepener and Birgit Weyel (Berlin: De Gruyter, 2018), 75–87, 80.

32 Cf. John 17:20f; Eph 4:5 and 1 Kor 12:27 etc.

33 Other religions have other pictures and symbols for transcendent communities. Cf. the concept of "umma" in muslim spirituality: Mahmoud Abdallah, "Religion, Gesellschaft und Moralwerte: Umma zwischen Heterogenität der Gegenwart und dem Traum von Einheit," *Ökumenische Rundschau* 65 (2016): 213–226.

34 Ulf Liedke, "Menschen. Leben. Vielfalt," *PTh* 101 (2012): 71–86, 81.

der Wahrnehmung behinderter Menschen) has been expressed. In light of the experience that people with mental diseases very often stay in special facilities, like psychiatric hospitals with specialized pastoral care, and that they do not remain embedded in their former environment, a dichotomic perspective has been wrongly established. People with mental disorders are no longer an individual, as a subject of the congregation, but they become an object of welfare. "Congregational participation from this background has been thought of most from the perspective of charity."[35] The well-meaning intention to help others, to offer welfare and support, causes an asymmetry that does not fit into the concept of Christian life as being the 'body of Christ'. Henning Luther has already pointed out this problem and claimed a change of view: "The others become an object of charitable welfare and pastoral care, as far as they have some deficits (passion/sin/error). The aim is the correction of the defects and the integration or rather reintegration of the other into the whole (of the congregation/the 'standards')."[36] Part of the twofold suppression in the charitable view is the intention to fade out one's own weakness and at the same time perceive the other only by his or her deficits.[37]

6.2 Congregations are Places for Interpretation of Life, Health and Illness

There are indeed many and multifold places in society where religion and spirituality can take place or just happen and experiences concerning health and illness can be interpreted,[38] not only in congregations. Lived religion is embedded in everyday life as part of culture, so religion and spirituality are not limited or restricted to worship or pastoral care. Wilhelm Gräb pointed out: "Religion belongs to the culture of everyday life in the way that religion with its symbols and rituals constitutes meaning in everyday life. Religion stands for meaning of life after all."[39] There are manifold constructions of life in between health and illness in

35 "Die kirchgemeindliche Teilhabe ist vor diesem Hintergrund maßgeblich unter dem Gesichtspunkt der Fürsorge gedacht worden." Liedke, "Menschen. Leben. Vielfalt," 80 (trans. Birgit Weyel).

36 Henning Luther, "Wahrnehmen und Ausgrenzen oder die doppelte Verdrängung. Zur Tradition des seelsorgerlich-diakonischen Blicks," *ThPr 23* (1988): 250–266, 261.

37 Cf. Liedke, "Menschen. Leben. Vielfalt," 71–86, 81.

38 Cf. Sabine Winkelmann, *Religiöse Deutung in schwerer Krankheit* (Berlin/Münster: Lit Verlag, 2016).

39 Cf. Wilhelm Gräb, *Religion als Deutung des Lebens. Perspektiven einer Praktischen Theologie gelebter Religion* (Gütersloh: Gütersloher Verlagshaus, 2006), 33. Own translation: "Religion gehört

daily communication with close friends and partners.[40] Even in the face of specialization in modern society, everyday life as a source for counselling and care might be out of view and has to be considered in poimenics. "There are many situations in the process of everyday life when spiritual care (Seelsorge) is possible and already happening. The conversations in pastoral care, which are conducted with the pastor, are associated with a culture of pastoral care conversation."[41]

Interpretation of illness (Krankheitsdeutung) is also a topic in the media, e.g. internet-platforms providing opportunities to exchange experiences by concerned people, and self-help books. Especially with regard to cancer, various books are also available.[42]

Congregations are places for interpretation of health and illness as well in pastoral care and worship, in congregational groups like choirs and in religious education. Congregations can benefit if they take these opportunities to contribute to health-related issues seriously.

---

so zur Alltagskultur, dass sie mit ihren Symbolen und Ritualen entscheidend am sinnhaften Aufbau der Alltagswelt beteiligt ist. Sie steht für den Sinn, den ihre Welt letzten Endes für die Menschen hat."

40 Cf. the network-analysis on religious communication ('meaning of life') of church-members in: Felix Roleder and Birgit Weyel, *Vernetzte Kirchengemeinde. Persönliche Beziehungen, religiöse Kommunikation, kirchliche Geselligkeit und zivilgesellschaftliche Beteiligung. Analysen zur Gesamtnetzwerkerhebung der V. Kirchenmitgliedschaftsuntersuchung der EKD* (Leipzig: Evangelische Verlagsanstalt, 2019).

41 Wolfgang Steck, "Der Ursprung der Seelsorge in der Alltagswelt," *ThZ 43* (1987): 175–183, 175. Own translation: "Es gibt ebenso viele Situationen im Ablauf des alltäglichen Lebens, in denen Seelsorge möglich ist und in denen sie auch praktiziert wird. Die Seelsorgegespräche, die mit dem Pfarrer geführt werden, ordnen sich in den Zusammenhang der seelsorgerlichen Gesprächskultur ein."

42 E.g. Christoph Schlingensief, *So schön wie hier kanns im Himmel gar nicht sein! Tagebuch einer Krebserkrankung* (Köln: Kiepenheuer & Witsch, 2009). Not only, but very often the guidebooks are published by celebrities.

I Religion and Health. An Overview

Michael Klessmann

Does Faith Heal?

Reflections on the Complex Relationship of Religion, Illness, and Health

1 Scenes to Introduce the Topic

The Gospel of Mark (5: 25–34) tells the story of a woman who suffers from bleeding for twelve years. Doctors could not help her and her illness just grew worse. She heard of the wandering rabbi and miracle healer named Jesus. She thought to herself, "if only I could touch his clothes, I would be made well" and pushed forward through the crowd that surrounded him. And then, as she touched him, she felt how her bleeding stopped, and at the same time, Jesus sensed strength leaving him. He discovered the woman, who was afraid that she had done something forbidden, and he said to her, "Your faith has healed you" (Mark 5: 34). Your faith has healed you physically but also in your relationships. The Greek verb σώζω used here means salvation from mortal danger, from the danger of illness, as well as figuratively the salvation from sin and guilt, from disturbed relationships. For this reason, healing is also regarded as a sign of the beginning of the Kingdom of God – the sick become physically healthy as well as being re-accepted into the community, which had excluded them because of their illness. To this extent, they are healed in a holistic way: physically and in terms of their social relationships.

The second scene: the Süddeutsche Zeitung reported in the 14 to 15 May 2016 issue in a whole page story about a journalist who multiple doctors agree has incurable cancer and only a few more weeks to live. Although the man does not really consider himself religious, he begins to pray and meditate intensively, and to the surprise of his doctors, the tumor completely disappears after a few weeks. Is this a spontaneous recovering or a healing through faith?

The third scene: a young woman who has two small children and is a member of my circle of friends falls ill with an incurable, inoperable lung tumor. She is a member of the church, speaks with the hospital chaplain when she goes to the hospital, prays and meditates more than before her illness, but is

Note: This lecture was originally held at the study day "Faith and Health in Cultural Context" at the University of Tuebingen on October 15, 2016.

https://doi.org/10.1515/9783110674217-002

not cured, and dies. It is normal that faith fails to make the sick healthy. Faith resulting in healing is the rare exception.

Ultimately, healers and healings using esoteric religious methods have existed for millennia. However, such healing methods and their promised results are viewed today as charlatanism and quackery and are regarded as dangerous and harmful because they deter the use of available conventional medical assistance.

Those who contemplate the relationship between faith, illness and healing would also do well to consider the following different contradictory aspects. Faith can contribute to healing and foster the interpersonal abilities of sick people. Faith often does not heal and can even harm. Moreover, there is a further variation: faith does not heal in a simple, causal sense, but allows for an altered approach to illness, a changed attitude toward illness and death. As Karl Barth put it, faith strengthens our "ability to be human" and therefore contains something healing.

2 On the Altered Relationship between Religion and Health in the Postmodern Age

From Antiquity to the Enlightenment, medicine and religion have been closely related. In Exodus 15: 26 it is exclaimed programmatically: "I am the Lord, who heals you." God wounds and bandages, he shatters and heals (Job 5:18). The doctor has a supporting role, but the actual healing power comes from God – or, as in the Hippocratic tradition, from nature. Therefore, it was long customary in simple medieval hospitals that the sick first confessed to a priest and had their sins forgiven: the person should be spiritually pure, freed from one's remoteness to God before it was considered reasonable to begin a medical treatment.

Since the Enlightenment, the systems of medicine and religion in Western societies have diverged. In the eyes of enlightened contemporaries it is no longer a God that miraculously heals in response to prayers and rituals, but rather the medical art of doctors. Scientific medicine increasingly identifies the physio-chemical causes of illness, treating them surgically or chemically (medicinally), and having enormous success. At the same time, criticism is voiced time and again that this scientific model of illness and health works in a reductionist way because bodily processes are separated from psychological, social and spiritual processes. However, there are other approaches:

- The persistent boom in alternative medicine (which includes a conglomerate of different methods) can be understood as a response to the ever-growing specialization within conventional medicine. Alternative medicine is a kind of holistic medicine in which the treatment is integrated into a relational-cosmos. Persons with organic disorders cannot be adequately understood and treated without taking into account their relationship with the environment, nature, fellow human beings, themselves, and (however it is understood) transcendence. When this happens, the treatment of a diseased organ can lead to the healing of the whole person.[1]

- Palliative care and hospice work have created a new perspective for holistic treatment and accompaniment of sick people. The WHO standards for palliative medicine explicitly specify that in addition to physical pain, psychological, social and spiritual problems and questions should also be given high priority in the treatment.
- The religious criticism, inspired by Sigmund Freud and widely accepted among medical professionals as well as psychologists well into the twentieth century, that says religion is an infantile projection of the humanly longing for a heavenly father figure, is hardly upheld today. The growing acceptance of Far Eastern religions and their practices has encouraged a different, so to say benevolent picture of religion. Religiosity and spirituality, the meaning dimension, have in a new way, become respectable and even worthy of research. Since then, religiosity has also been regarded as a resource whose capabilities are used in life and disease management.
- Since the late 1980s, there has also been increasingly more and explicit research on the connection between religion and health, primarily in the USA, but also in Europe. The surprising and sometimes contradictory research results have even convinced religious critics that one cannot simply ignore this topic.
- Finally, the widespread systemic orientation within the field of social sciences has contributed to a new reputation for this topic. In systemic thinking, one assumes that everything that is part of a system also has an effect. Religious beliefs – systemic psychologists speak of God constructs – are constituents of individual, familial and social systems, and as such are effective in every case. However, this effectiveness can be constructive as well as destructive.[2]

With this changed discussion, two branches of tradition are coming back together that have been closely linked for centuries. On the one hand, there are

1 Cf. Josef Mayer-Scheu and Rudolf Kautsky, eds., *Vom Behandeln zum Heilen. Die vergessene Dimension im Krankenhaus* (Wien/Göttingen: Herder, 1980).

2 Cf. Christoph Morgenthaler, *Systemische Seelsorge* (Stuttgart: Kohlhammer, 1999), 76–95.

the abundance of concrete healing practices that have existed for thousands of years in all cultures (care of wounds, knowledge of herbs, massage techniques, etc.) that always involved a religious dimension, because disease was primarily viewed as disturbance of a comprehensive system of life and wholeness. For a long time, healing was understood not only as physical restitution, but above all as restoration of the lost balance in the relationship to God, and consequently to the world, fellow human beings and oneself. Jesus first forgives the sins of the paralytic. His healing is the result and expression of forgiveness, that is, the restored order with God and with life as a whole. Salvation (shalom), which God gives, will be anticipated and symbolized (therefore fragmented) in the experience of healing.

On the other hand, however, we have to work from the assumption of an "independence of bodily phenomena."[3] Not every illness has a (causally understood) psychological or spiritual dimension. Rapidly growing tumors, such as brain tumors or pancreatic cancer, elicit intolerable pressure on those affected, especially when suggesting that lifestyle and emotions could contribute to the illness, or altered behavior could have even prevented the illness. These negative sides of a holistic perspective on health and disease must be considered.

Note regarding terminology: I use the term *religion* for "a symbol system…, referring to 'another reality,'"[4] a system of faiths, values, traditions, rituals and roles, which have found an organizational structure through the formation of religious communities. I understand *religiosity or faith* as a personal-subjective internal position of those who belong to a religious community, a religious system. *Spirituality* is related to such a religiosity, but it is less connected to a religious system, more pluralized, and therefore to a large degree personality-specific. Spirituality is characterized by experience, that is, through a holistic form of recognition including thinking, feeling and motivation to act, which refers to a reality that exceeds the individual self.

3 Research Results on the Relationship between Religion and Health

In the USA there have been remarkable research findings regarding the connection between religion and health for many years. One summary study says, "Over

---

3 Cf. Isolde Karle, "Die Sehnsucht nach Heil und nach Heilung in der kirchlichen Praxis," in *Krankheitsdeutung in der postsäkularen Gesellschaft*, eds. Günter Thomas and Isolde Karle (Stuttgart: Kohlhammer, 2009): 550.

4 Hans-Peter Hasenfratz, *Religion – was ist das?* (Freiburg: Herder, 2002), 9.

1,200 American studies show a positive statistical link between physical health and personal beliefs, which can be interpreted as causal. This means that those who believe are healthy, have more coping strategies and enjoy a higher level of satisfaction for life, and even a higher life expectancy."[5] The connection between religiosity and mental disorder or mental disease is also described as clearly positive. Especially with regard to widespread depression, it can be asserted that a strong religiosity is associated with fewer depressive symptoms. Prominent American researchers such as Harold Koenig and Herbert Benson have supported the thesis, stating, "Religiosity is always associated with better health."[6] Even the magazine "Psychologie heute" jumped on the bandwagon and in 2005 published an article entitled "Faith and health. Why hope can heal."[7] This article summarizes a large number of American studies on the subject accordingly: "religious people are less likely to be hospitalized, have lower blood pressure, and appear to be better protected against cardiovascular diseases."[8]

A critical review of these one-sidedly positive results was not long in coming about and seems absolutely necessary to me considering that the cultural background of American religiosity is so fundamentally different from European religiosity, so that such results cannot simply be transferred to our Western European context. From the perspective of psychology of religion, it is often pointed out that the constructs of religiosity and health are very difficult to operationalize because they are so highly multifactorial that the research results often do not do justice to the complexity of the subject matter.[9]

Possible harmful connections between religiosity and health that may result from strict religious socializations (uncertainty, fears, anger, or rage) have not been systematically researched, and are based more on anecdotal reports.[10]

From a theological point of view, legitimate criticism says that faith cannot be functionalized. Any reckoning with the healing effects of faith means its perversion. The belief in God, in an omnipotent reality does not aim to achieve anything, but rather to honor God and identify humans as God's creation.

---

5 Simone Ehm and Michael Utsch, "Glaube und Gesundheit. Historische Zusammenhänge und aktuelle Befunde," *EZW-Texte* 181 (2005): 5–16, 7.

6 Herbert Benson, *Heilung durch Glauben* (München: Heyne, 1997), 210. Similar: Harold George Koenig, *Is Religion Good for your Health?* (New York/London: Haworth Pastoral Press, 1997).

7 *Psychologie Heute* 32 (2005).

8 *Psychologie Heute* 32 (2005): 21–22.

9 Cf. Marion Schowalter and Sebastian Murken, "Religion und psychische Gesundheit – empirische Zusammenhänge komplexer Konstrukte," in *Einführung in die Religionspsychologie*, eds. Christian Henning, Sebastian Murken and Erich Nestler (Paderborn: UTB, 2003): 138–162.

10 Cf. Michael Utsch, *Religiöse Fragen in der Psychotherapie* (Stuttgart: Kohlhammer, 2005), 159–161.

The research results in secularized Europe are much more reserved and skeptical. The German religious psychologist Bernhard Grom summarized the debate about the connection between religion and health as follows: "Experts broadly agree that attending worship services and positive forms of personal religiosity are statistically linked to subjective well-being and mental health. This relationship is statistically weak to moderate, but significant and very likely also causal."[11]

The positive impact that a religious attitude towards health, or health management has, or should have, is attributed to a number of factors, which formulated as hypotheses guide the research.[12]

- A *behavioral hypothesis* assumes that through behavioral rules regarding diet, sexuality, etc., a certain religious affiliation can have a direct impact on health. This sounds obvious. Those who due to their religious affinity do not smoke or drink (Mormons, Jehovah's Witnesses, etc.) and altogether lead a relatively regulated life, undoubtedly live healthier than most other contemporaries do.
- The *cohesion hypothesis* highlights the instrumental importance of trusting relationships and a supportive network within a religious community. Social cohesion in pietistic circles is often very tight, as is the social control. Church communities, in which true trust, reciprocal support and participation are experienced, contribute to the health of their members in a way that should not be underestimated. Social support is also known to be a stress buffer,[13] but at the same time, social control can also create new stress.
- The *coherence hypothesis* suggests that religious explanations for critical life events provide a psychological advantage because those affected do not feel helpless, but rather can understand the events as meaningful. Interpretation, understood as cognitive structuring of an unmanageable world, makes trust possible and thus potentially results in more serenity, which in turn can have a positive effect on healing or disease management.
- Similarly, the *coping hypothesis* refers to the improved ability to cope with crisis situations. Faith provides safety and security. Prayer meditation offer

11 Bernhard Grom, "Wie froh macht die Frohbotschaft? Religiosität, subjektives Wohlbefinden und psychische Gesundheit," *WzM* 54 (2002): 196–204, 199.

12 Concerning the following issues cf. Sebastian Murken, "Ungesunde Religiosität – Entscheidungen der Psychologie?" in *Kritik an Religionen*, eds. Gritt Maria Klinkhammer, Steffen Rink and Tobias Frick (Marburg: Diagonal-Verlag, 1997): 157–159.

13 Cf. Sabine Allwinn, "Krankheitsbewältigung als individueller, interaktiver und sozialer Prozess," in *Psychosoziale Dienste und Seelsorge im Krankenhaus*, eds. Christoph Schneider-Harpprecht and Sabine Allwinn (Göttingen: Vandenhoeck & Ruprecht, 2005): 42.

ways of entrusting oneself and one's own worries to God: to let oneself enter into a trusting relationship and to feel secure in it can activate hope and serenity in a similar manner.[14]

- The *self-worth hypothesis* says that the belief of being accepted, justified and loved by God strengthens self-esteem, which in turn contributes to improved health – while self-doubt and self-uncertainty rather tend to have a negative effect.
- There is also a *stress reduction hypothesis*. Meditation research has found that meditation initiates a relaxation process that can be clearly identified in the brain. In fact, "meditative practices lower the heart rate, reduce skin conductance and soothe metabolism."[15] Also, especially if one is in a depressive mood, or suffers from anxiety and sleep disorder, meditation enables one to let go of negative feelings and reduces brooding.
- *Finally, there is also a placebo hypothesis.*[16] A positive expectation of a medication or a curative treatment can lead to strong results; doctors have known this for a long time. The religious acceptance of God's love and salvation, combined with reconciliation with one's own destiny, can, like a placebo, promote inner peace and balance, thus contributing to recovery or better means of coping with disease.

Two critical remarks at this point:

First off, as criteria for the measurement of religious orientation, self-reports from people (such as how often they attend worship, how often they pray, and if they consider themselves faithful or religious) are used in the majority of the studies. It is known that such self-reports are notoriously unreliable, and they say little about the kind of religiosity. Already in the 1950s, the American religious psychologist Gordon Allport proposed the distinction between an extrinsically and intrinsically motivated religiosity. This is, on the one hand, some people regularly go to church because their family and neighbourhood do so, and not being seen there would be socially disadvantageous. On the other hand, some are indifferent to what those in their surroundings think, having an inner mission and believing in God, a divine power. But how can these differences be identified?

14 Cf. Harald Walach, "Spiritualität als Ressource. Chancen und Probleme eines neuen Forschungsfeldes," *EZW-Texte* 181 (2005): 17–40, especially 27–29.

15 Ulrich Schnabel, *Die Vermessung des Glaubens*, Vol. 2 (München: Pantheon Verlag, 2010), 236.

16 Schnabel, *Die Vermessung des Glaubens*, 45–47.

Secondly, one also has to take the possible downsides of religion into consideration.[17] Unfortunately, there are clearly negative correlations between religiosity and every day behavior. For example, there is an alarming correlation between religiosity and prejudice.[18] In addition, within religious communities, one can also observe exclusion and intolerance against minorities, cognitive rigidity, and an increase in negative emotions such as fear of punishment or self-condemnation, so that certain forms of religiosity can become a risk or a factor of vulnerability.[19] Religiosity combined with anxiety, feelings of guilt and pressure from the outside produces new fears, depressive states and physical ailments.[20] How does this fit together with the supposed healing factor of faith?

4 Models of Classification

Individual reports of experiences and the multitude of empirical studies must remain contested when it is not possible to develop convincing model-concepts that can theoretically reconstruct the interdependence of faith, religiosity or spirituality on the one hand and health or disease management on the other hand. I would like to introduce two such models. The first well-known model developed by Aaron Antonovsky is called salutogenesis. The second model, known as the concept of self-regulation, was designed by Ronald Grossart-Maticek and validated in long-term prospective studies.

Antonovsky[21] assumes, what every human knows from his or her own experience, that health and illness are not mutually exclusive states, but are connected to each other in a flexible continuum. What moves people on this continuum more toward health or more toward illness? This is a central question to which Antonovsky developed the following answer. Everyone is constantly confronted with stressful life and environmental situations, or so-called stressors. Whether these stressors have pathogenic, neutral or even healthy

---

17 Cf. Bernhard Grom, *Religionspsychologie* (München/Göttingen: Kösel-Verlag, 1992), 374–376.

18 Cf. Beate Küpper and Andreas Zick, "Riskanter Glaube. Religiosität und Abwertung," in *Deutsche Zustände. Folge 4*, ed. Wilhelm Heitmeyer (Frankfurt: Suhrkamp, 2006): 179–188.

19 Cf. Gunther Klosinksi, ed., *Religion als Chance oder Risiko* (Bern: Verlag Hans Huber, 1994) and Sebastian Murken, *Gottesbeziehung und psychische Gesundheit* (Münster/New York: Waxmann, 1998). Summarizing his study, Murken points to the aspect that negative correlation between religiosity and mental health is far easier to establish than positive correlation!

20 Cf. Judith Lindner, "Einflüsse von Religiosität und Vergebung auf die psychische Gesundheit," *WzM* 68 (2016): 360–371.

21 Cf. Heiko Waller, *Gesundheitswissenschaft*, Vol. 2 (Stuttgart/Berlin: Kohlhammer, 1996), 17–19.

effects depends on the one hand on the strengths and nature of the stressors, and on the other hand on the resistance resources that persons are provided with through their genetic equipment or rather those which their environment has given them. These include physical resources (resilience of the immune system), psychological resources (mental stability and flexibility combined with intelligence and knowledge), material resources (work, housing, income), and psychosocial resources (interpersonal relationships, being socially integrated and connected, the possibility of support, exchange and help).

The various resources are held together and are activated by a central subjective competence, which Antonovsky calls "coherence." Coherence refers to the feeling that there is connection and meaning in life, that life is not subject to a fate that cannot be influenced.[22] The sense of coherence describes a spiritual attitude that is characterized as follows:

> My world is largely understandable, harmonious, ordered; also, problems and burdens that I experience, I can see in a larger context and therefore deal with. I have resources that I can mobilize to master life, especially when facing problems and crises. (Antonovsky calls Job an example of a person with a sense of coherence because even in the most difficult situations, he maintains his trust in the righteousness of God.)

The antithesis to coherence is the state of demoralization. It is precisely from this negative pole that the concept becomes clear. A patient in a psychiatric clinic once told me: "I have never had my life under control; I never knew where I belonged." One can easily imagine how distressing and agonizing such a feeling towards life is.

An integral part of the sense of coherence is, of course, the worldview of a person, one's life philosophy, religiosity, and faith. This does not refer to religious or confessional affiliation, but rather to a life perspective that influences and shapes understanding, feeling and behavior. What this means can be illustrated through a series of questions, which, I think, everyone asks themselves at some point or even several times in their lives. These questions include: How does reality confront me as a whole? How do I perceive life? – As a capricious destiny whose unpredictability I'm hopelessly exposed to so that I can only react with fear and uncertainty? As cruel ruthlessness to which I can only depressively resign? As a rigorous challenge that drives me to the highest accomplishments and efforts, but to which I never really do justice? As an ultimately loving, supportive base in which I can feel trusted and release myself? As encouragement for love of one's self and of the other?

---

22 Aaron Antonovsky, *Health, Stress and Coping* (San Francisco: Jossey-Bass, 1979), 123–125.

Depending on one's attitude towards life, the sense of coherence is influenced and thereby also influences the resources of resistance with regard to illness and health.

Ronald Grossarth-Maticek, a professor of social medicine from Heidelberg, developed a similar approach with the concept of self-regulation.[23] Grossarth-Maticek supports a systemic-interactive medicine that assumes that all genetic-physiological factors contributing to illness or health are superimposed and influenced to a high degree through emotional-cognitive control and evaluation mechanisms. Behind this is an anthropology in which the human appears "as a highly complex, interactive, socio-psycho-biological system which strives towards competent desire, well-being, inner and outer security and fulfillment. The human is an emotional-cognitive, actively controlled, self-regulated, yet interactively dependent system that is constantly creating conditions, expressing and satisfying needs in his or her own body and in the environment."[24] Many people lost the ability for active and flexible self-regulation, whether by early discouraging social experiences, biographical shock-experiences, patronizing structures in the world of work, or a highly specialized medicine that makes the individual into an object of their intervention through mono-causal explanatory approaches. With the help of a so-called autonomy training designed by Grossart-Maticek, the ability for a constructive self-regulation based on needs and an appropriate relationship between closeness and distance can be restored or strengthened.

A component of self-regulation is, according to Grossarth-Maticek, the experienced God-human relationship. The author assumes that every person has such a relationship (God understood as a source of love, communication, and helpful order),[25] be it engaging, rejecting, or even indifferent in nature. In any case, the experienced God-human relationship has an impact on motivation and action, and therefore indirectly also on well-being and health. This is because, depending on its individual manifestation, the God-human relationship conveys, love, trust and hope, or fear, the feeling of heteronomity and restrained ability to love.[26]

From a theological point of view, such classification models have been criticized in that the relationship between religiosity and health is seen as purely functional and thereby excludes the question of content and truth. This

---

23 Ronald Grossarth-Maticek, *Selbstregulation, Autonomie und Gesundheit* (Berlin/New York: De Gruyter, 2003).

24 Grossarth-Maticek, *Selbstregulation, Autonomie und Gesundheit*, 30.

25 Grossarth-Maticek, *Selbstregulation, Autonomie und Gesundheit*, 22.

26 Cf. Grossarth-Maticek, *Selbstregulation, Autonomie und Gesundheit*, 283–285.

observation is correct, but limited in its range. New Testament healing stories, for example, also show the curative effect of faith in a non-qualified way: "Your faith has saved you," as I quoted from Mark 5:34, and this is said in many other places. The New Testament scholar Ulrich Luz interprets the parallel passage in Matthew 9:22 with his own words as "Faith is something active, a venture of unlimited trust in Jesus. On such ventures, however ambiguous, Jesus answers and promises God's help … "[27]

In light of such an interpretation, two perspectives of explanation exist. They belong together and complement one another, but must be distinguished. On the one hand, the effectiveness of faith is emphasized: Faith as the human's act of trust in God or Jesus as the miracle worker, as the incarnation of the "human-border-transgression",[28] rescues, helps, makes healthy. This corresponds to what the coherence or self-regulation hypotheses say, stating similarly that forces are released (can they be called self-healing forces?[29]) that apparently develop a healing effect. On the other hand, the unavailability of this event is emphasized. In the healing stories, Jesus, the miracle worker, establishes the faith of the person seeking help, by speaking to them. Therefore, it is clear that the healing effect of faith is God's work; the revelation of the Holy One, in a sense, releases faith and healing. The impact of faith is not calculable nor can it be sued for. On an empirical level, this theological statement corresponds to the fact that the healing effect of religiosity and faith in concrete individual cases is never directly and monocausally verifiable. Whether the healing of the journalist cited at the beginning is due to his praying and meditation remains pure speculation. Therefore, healing through faith does not represent something that those can count on, for which they can plan. There always remains just one last subsequent interpretation (some talk of faith healing and others of spontaneous healing), which has a certain probability from the statistical middle – no more and no less.

Both levels of interpretation, the theological and the empirical, do not only not contradict each other, but they need each other. A theological perspective that does not at least rudimentarily try to look for empirical realization possibilities hardly appears credible. Conversely, an empirical perspective,

27 Ulrich Luz, *Evangelisch-Katholischer Kommentar zum Neuen Testament Tb. 2 – Das Evangelium nach Matthäus (Mt 8–17)* (Zürich/Neukirchen: Benzinger/Neukirchener, 1990): 53.
28 Cf. Gerd Theißen, *Urchristliche Wundergeschichten*, Vol. 5 (Gütersloh: Gueterslоher Verlagshaus, 1987), 142.
29 Cf. Klaus Berger, "Biblisches Christentum als Heilungsreligion," in *Heilung – Energie – Geist. Heilung zwischen Wissenschaft, Religion und Geschäft*, eds. Werner Heinz Ritter and Bernhard Wolf (Göttingen: Vandenhoeck & Ruprecht, 2005): 226–246, 230.

be it religious psychology or medical-psychosomatic, does well when it takes the theological reservations of the unavailability of healing seriously and remembers its limits.

5 A Different Perspective on Faith, Illness, and Health, Healing and Salvation

We live in a time where health has become one of the highest virtues and goals. The physician and theologian Manfred Lütz writes sarcastically, "If there is anything at all on the altar today, which is worshiped and acknowledged with every kind of sweat-producing sacrifice, it is health."[30] We are to produce these sacrifices through multiple measures: through awareness of healthy nutrition, through exercise and fitness, through stimulating social contacts and balanced emotionality. A positive religious attitude, called spirituality, can through meditation, fasting, pilgrimages, etc., certainly contribute to health.

With such an understanding, both concept of health and that of faith have been curtailed and distorted. As a final point, I would like to elaborate on this.

With the World Health Organization's definition of health from 1946, we have been left with an ambiguous legacy. Accordingly, health is "a state of complete physical, mental and social well-being." Such a definition had a pioneering function directly after the catastrophe of the Second World War. Not only physical, but also psychological and social factors were clearly responsible for illness and health and required appropriate socio-political measures. At the same time, with this definition something like an expectation of entitlement in terms of health was created in Western societies: exaggerated expectations for complete well-being, for salvation – such unrealistic expectations can never be met.

This becomes clear when I contrast this understanding with two other concepts of health. The first has a systemic perspective. It says, "healthy is a person who with or without demonstrable or for him perceptible deficiencies of his corporeality, with or without the help of others, finds, develops and maintains an equilibrium, which enables him to live a meaningful life and attain life goals

30 Werner Heinz Ritter, "Heilung, Energie, Geist als wissenschaftliche Herausforderung," in *Heilung – Energie – Geist. Heilung zwischen Wissenschaft, Religion und Geschäft*, eds. Werner Heinz Ritter and Bernhard Wolf (Göttingen: Vandenhoeck & Ruprecht, 2005): 15–30, 16.

based on the unfolding of his personal assets and life plans within his limitations so that he can say: my life, my illness, my death."[31]

Here it is noteworthy that life as a whole, but especially illness and health are understood as open processes of equilibrium and relationships. Social frameworks, social interaction and subjective feelings form a vulnerable network. When one succeeds in balancing these different factors alone or with the help of others, then one can call oneself healthy, even if there is a restriction or handicap. Not only the limitations come into view, but also the resources. And at the same time, the fundamental limitation of life must be taken into account: my life, my illness, my death.

Ivan Illich (1926–2002), a philosopher, theologian and medical critic who became famous in the 1970s said, "Health is the ability to adapt to changing milieus, to grow up, to age, to recover in case of injury, to suffer, and to await death in peace .... The deliberately lived fragility, individuality and social openness of the human make the experience of pain, illness and death an integral part of life. The ability to manage these three things autonomously is the foundation of health."[32] In this concept, health has to do with the ability to cope with life – and coping with life means always coping with pain, suffering, limitations and losses. The emphasis is on limitation. Therefore, the individual and social illusion of omnipotence, to be able to do everything, to heal everything, to overcome all boundaries – and conventional medicine nurtures this illusion with their successes – should be exposed and one should live according to the ethics of limitations.

In such a context, one cannot simply functionalize and exploit the faith, the religiosity or spirituality of a person. Faith, as I understand it, means to know that one is carried by and dependent on one greater than oneself. I owe my life not to my achievements and myself, but to a greater one, call it God or the divine, the holy, the transcendence. To trust this greater one, benevolent and turning to us in all sorts of daily hardships on the one hand, demanding and threatening on the other, means to see oneself as essentially limited, dependent and fragmented. We do not have our lives in our hands, we do not create it ourselves, we do not create identity, meaning and also health ourselves, rather they are given to us. We owe our lives, mourning and petitionary prayers in light of damaged or limited life and thanks for improvements and healings are fundamental forms of religious communication. In this context, it is necessary to be prepared for illnesses and be aware of our mortality and to accept them as part of created life when they occur.

---

31 Fritz Hartmann, "Krank oder bedingt gesund?," *MMG* 11 (1986): 170–179, 172.

32 Ivan Illich, *Nemesis der Medizin* (Reinbek: Rowohlt, 1977), 309 and 311.

The contribution of the Christian faith to the debate about the connection between faith and health, in my opinion, is not made with the intention to functionalize faith for health and thus to continue to support the health and performance ideology of capitalist societies, but rather with the opposite intention, namely, to introduce a "moderate" understanding of health which is based on relationships.

The English psychoanalyst Donald Winnicott described how holding and being held constitute one of the most fundamental experiences for parents and children. A child must feel that he or she is held in a literal and figurative sense, for better or worse. More and more, this process is becoming an image for me of what is meant by faith: This feeling of being held and cared for, also as an adult and elderly person, by other people, family members, friends, and to sense a greater unconditional and indefinite care in those limited and fragmented forms of being held. Anyone who knows this will also be more comfortable with the evils of illness because he or she feels that his or her value as a person does not depend on the illness and its possible limitations.

In this way, the difference between salvation and healing comes into view. I would translate the term salvation as, with faith in God, one is absolutely valued and recognized, independent of his or her life situation, actual health or disease status. In services of blessing and annointing, this appreciation is promised to humans in a sensuous form. For some, this may sound like utopia, a vision, a longing worth living for. Others may actually experience this salvation in short moments. Even if the healing is not complete, if limitations and pain do not disappear, this notion of salvation in the sense of unconditional acknowledgment remains and makes it easier to hold on to hope in face of illness and restrictions.

In this context, the theologian and physician Dietrich Ritschl proposed the metaphor of "Athens" and "Jerusalem".[33] Athens represents the ancient ideal of the Greeks, the healthy, beautiful, strong, athletic, young man – conforming to contemporary ideal of health. Jerusalem, on the other hand, refers to the broken, suffering and crucified Jesus of Nazareth. The metaphor of Jerusalem reflects a different concept of health; not the WHO's full-bodied one, but rather one that describes health as the ability to endure and cope with experiences of pain, illness and fragility in communion with others. With this, the health policy perspective changes fundamentally. We do not allow a concept of health to be prescribed and we do not ask about the functional contribution of religiosity and faith in order to reach an even better and more comprehensive condition.

---

33 Cf. Dietrich Ritschl, "Gesundheit: Gnade oder Rechtsanspruch," in *Konzepte. Ökumene, Medizin, Ethik*, ed. Dietrich Ritschl (München: Kaiser, 1986): 266–271.

Conversely, based on Christian tradition, we develop a human image[34] from which perceptions of health and illness are to be created in critical analysis with contemporary concepts. The moment of the relationship to others, to environment and transcendence, and the moment of passivity and receptivity, of need and dependence, of acceptance of the fragmentary as an integral part of the healthy person must also play a major role in this. Only as a side comment, let me mention the weight of resistance and of struggling against the disease. It is my impression that the medical system as a whole provokes this well enough. What we urgently need is the acceptance of the fragmentary, of that which is not successful. It is most likely that the connection between Christian faith and such an understanding of health can hardly be empirically verified, and yet its contribution to humanizing health care could be considerable.

34 Cf. Dietrich Ritschl, "Was ist der Mensch – in Krankheit und Gesundheit? Anthropologische Ansätze verschiedener Krankheits- und Gesundheitsverständnisse," *WzM* 51 (1999): 396–410.

Christian Zwingmann and Constantin Klein

Religion and Health from the View of Psychology of Religion

Empirical Results – Possible Pathways – Cultural Context

1 Introduction

This chapter gives an overview of the current state of socio-scientific research on the relation between religiosity and health discussing the possible pathways from religious beliefs and behavior to health. Research on this topic has been increasing since the early 1990s, particularly in the United States. For instance, a literature review using the database MEDLINE (search terms: "religio*" & "health") showed an average of only 247 results per year from 1986 to 1990, but 1,728 results per year from 2014 to 2018. Therefore, the annual number of publications has nearly multiplied sevenfold since the early 1990s. Due to this enormous increase of studies, our article focuses primarily on existing reviews and meta-analyses.

In the field of religion and health, the term "religiosity" is usually understood rather substantially than functionally and includes the belief in a transcendent reality.[1] "Religiosity" often speaks to a specific semantic domain, particularly those associated with Christianity. Many studies highlight the importance of an intrinsically motivated religiosity which means that religiosity has an end in and of itself while playing an important role in someone's personal life.[2] Intrinsic religiosity can thus be described as the "centrality of religiosity in one's life."[3] Besides the term "religiosity", the relatively vague term "spirituality" has become very popular in recent years.[4] The relation between

1 Cf. Helfried Moosbrugger, Christian Zwingmann and Dirk Frank, "Psychologische Aspekte von Religiosität," in *Religiosität, Persönlichkeit und Verhalten. Beiträge zur Religionspsychologie*, eds. Helfried Moosbrugger, Christian Zwingmann and Dirk Frank (Münster: Waxmann, 1996): 3–8.

2 Cf. Gordon W. Allport and J. Michael Ross, "Personal religious orientation and prejudice," *Journal of Personality and Social Psychology 5* (1967): 432–443.

3 Cf. Stefan Huber, *Zentralität und Inhalt: Ein neues multidimensionales Messmodell der Religiosität* (Opladen: Leske & Budrich, 2003).

4 Cf. Harold G. Koenig, "Concerns about measuring 'spirituality' in research," *Journal of Nervous and Mental Disease 196* (2008): 349–355.

https://doi.org/10.1515/9783110674217-003

religiosity and spirituality is discussed controversially.[5] In the literature, spirituality is primarily understood as the wider concept which contains distinct "religiosities" as specific sets of beliefs and practices of a particular tradition. In this article, "religiosity" shall primarily express the subjective belief in something transcendent which has not necessarily been institutionalized; therefore, the meanings of "religiosity" and "spirituality" converge widely.

Most reviews of the research literature focus on studies from the Anglo-American context, in particular from the U.S., and insofar this article is based on such reviews it might be subject to a particular cultural bias. Both religiosity and health are disparate, multidimensional constructs. In many studies, however, only one dimension of religiosity or of health was operationalized, and sometimes studies are limited by the fact that only single-item measures were used. As a consequence, such studies tend to result in heterogeneous findings. Furthermore, as the literature reviews reveal, many studies are only cross-sectional so that causal conclusions cannot be drawn. Longitudinal studies and explicit testing of theoretical models can be supportive; however much like experimental studies, such articles are rare for the topic of religiosity and health.

2 Religiosity and Mental Health

Most studies show positive associations between religiosity and mental health. In particular an intrinsically motivated, personally relevant, constructive-positive religiosity is rarely associated with discomfort and uneasiness. Relations between religiosity and diverse dimensions of mental health are detailed below.

2.1 Subjective Well-being

Subjective well-being is a multidimensional construct embracing cognitive and emotional components. There is a great number of studies about relations between religiosity and several indicators of well-being which have repeatedly been examined in research reviews and meta-analyses. Since the 1990s, the tenor of these publications is almost the same: There are more positive than negative associations or zero-correlations in non-clinical and clinical samples.

5 Brian J. Zinnbauer and Kenneth I. Pargament, "Religiousness and spirituality," in *Handbook of the psychology of religion and spirituality*, eds. Raymond Paloutzian and Crystal L. Park (New York: Guilford, 2005): 21–42.

If all studies of interest are subsumed, they result in a (mostly weak) positive correlation.[6] Positive associations are especially observable when measures of intrinsic religiosity and personal devotion are used and when well-being is not assessed negatively in terms of low burden but positively in terms of desirable mental states.[7] Specific positive indicators of subjective well-being which have been investigated are: life satisfaction, meaning, internal control attribution, optimism, self-esteem, personal growth, and marital stability and satisfaction, to name a few.[8]

2.2 Depression and Suicide

An impressive meta-analysis including 147 relevant studies indicates that intrinsic religiosity and religious commitment and practice are associated with lower levels of depression as well as less depressive symptoms. The observation is of a medium size and robust effect.[9] According to this meta-analysis and an extensive longitudinal study by Kendler, Gardner, and Prescott,[10] there is an

6 Cf. C. Daniel Batson, Patricia Schoenrade and W. Larry Ventis, *Religion and the individual. A social-psychological perspective* (New York: Oxford University Press, 1993); Harold G. Koenig and David B. Larson, "Religion and mental health. Evidence for an association," *International Review of Psychiatry 13* (2001): 67–78; John M. Salsman et al., "A meta-analytic approach to examining the correlation between religion/spirituality and mental health in cancer," *Cancer 121* (2015): 3769–3778; Harold G. Koenig, Michael E. McCullough and David B. Larson, *Handbook of religion and health* (New York: Oxford University Press, 2001); Harold G. Koenig, Dana King and Verna B. Carson, *Handbook of religion and health.* 2nd edition (New York: Oxford University Press, 2012).

7 Cf. Michael J. Donahue, "Intrinsic and extrinsic religiousness: Review and meta-analysis," *Journal of Personality and Social Psychology 48* (1985): 55–67; Charles H. Hackney and Glenn S. Sanders, "Religiosity and mental health: A meta-analysis of recent studies," *Journal for the Scientific Study of Religion 42* (2003): 43–55.

8 Cf. Bernhard Grom, "Religiosität – psychische Gesundheit – subjektives Wohlbefinden: Ein Forschungsüberblick," in *Religiosität: Messverfahren und Studien zu Gesundheit und Lebensqualität. Neue Beiträge zur Religionspsychologie*, eds. Christian Zwingmann and Helfried Moosbrugger (Münster: Waxmann, 2004): 187–214; Koenig et al., *Handbook of religion and health*; Koenig et al., *Handbook of religion and health.* 2nd edition.

9 Cf. Timothy B. Smith, Michael E. McCullough and Justin Poll, "Religiousness and depression: Evidence for a main effect and the moderating influence of stressful live events," *Psychological Bulletin* 129 (2003): 614–636.

10 Cf. Kenneth S. Kendler, Charles O. Gardner and Carol A. Prescott, "Clarifying the relationship between religiosity and psychiatric illness: The impact of covariates and the specificity of buffering effects," *Twin Research and Human Genetics 2* (1999): 137–144.

inverse relationship between stronger religious beliefs and activities as compared to the risk and potential for manifestation of major depression. Additionally, the degree of suicidal tendencies is somewhat lower among religiously affiliated and actively committed persons.[11] Furthermore, religious coping strategies seem to provide some protection against depressive tendencies among terminally ill, bereaved, and caregivers.[12] Finally, therapeutic interventions including religious elements have shown to be successful in the treatment of depressive patients.[13]

2.3 Substance Abuse

In most studies, there is a slightly negative correlation between religiosity and the use and abuse of alcohol.[14] Church attendance and intrinsic religiosity can be considered to be relatively strong predictors of lower rates of substance abuse among pupils and students for example.[15] In this context, the effect of intrinsic religiosity is stronger than the effects of self-esteem and meaning-making, but weaker than the effects of parenting style and peer

---

11 Cf. Raphael Bonelli and Harold G. Koenig, "Mental disorders, religion and spirituality 1990 to 2010: A systematic evidence-based review," *Journal of Religion and Health 52* (2013): 657–673; Bernhard Grom, "Suizidalität und Religiosität," in *Suizidforschung und Suizidprävention am Ende des 20. Jahrhunderts. Theologische, epidemiologische, ökonomische, therapeutische Aspekte*, eds. Manfred Wolfersdorf and Christoph Franke (Regensburg: Roderer, 2000): 19–35; Jan Neeleman and Glenn Lewis, "Suicide, religion, and socioeconomic conditions. An ecological study in 26 countries," *Journal of Epidemiology and Community Health 53* (1999): 204–210.

12 Cf. Thomas G. Plante and Naveen K. Sharma, "Religious faith and mental health outcomes," in *Faith and health. Psychological perspectives*, eds. Thomas G. Plante and Allen C. Sherman (New York: Guilford, 2001): 240–261.

13 Cf. Michael E. McCullough, "Research on religion-accomodative counseling: Review and meta-analysis," *Journal of Counseling Psychology 46* (1999): 92–98.

14 Cf. Bonelli and Koenig, "Mental disorders, religion and spirituality," 657–673; Cynthia Geppert, Michael Bogenschutz and William Miller, "Development of a bibliography on religion, spirituality and addictions," *Drug and Alcohol Review 26* (2007): 389–395; Harold G. Koenig, *Spirituality in patient care: Why, how, when and what* (Philadelphia: Templeton Foundation Press, 2002).

15 Cf. e.g. Riia K. Luhtanen and Jennifer Crocker, "Alcohol use in college students: Effects of level of self-esteem, narcissism and contingencies of self-worth," *Psychology and Addictive Behaviors 19* (2005): 99–103; Thomas A. Wills, Alison M. Yaeger and James M. Sandy, "Buffering effect of religiosity for adolescent substance use," *Psychology of Addictive Behaviors 17* (2003): 24–31. Cf. Julie E. Yonker, Chelsea A. Schnabelrauch and Laura G. DeHaan, "The relationship between spirituality and religiosity on psychological outcomes in adolescents and emerging adults: A meta-analytic review," *Journal of Adolescence 35* (2012): 299–314.

attitudes.[16] In the treatment of addicts, higher religiosity seems to be associated with better coping and more resilience.[17] Several programmes for the treatment of addictions include particular spiritual elements. A common example is the 12 step programme of Alcoholics Anonymous.[18] Whether these elements are necessary for successful therapy remains unclear for the time being.[19]

2.4 Schizophrenia

Religiosity is probably no etiological factor of disorders of the schizophrenia spectrum, but might affect the symptomatic expressions of a schizophrenic disorder. Religiously socialized schizophrenic patients, for instance, seem to experience religious delusions more frequently than profane delusions.[20] However, this association is not very strong and seems to depend on the sociocultural context.[21] Although some studies indicate that, on the average, schizophrenia and other psychoses seem to exhibit higher religiosity than well-adjusted religious devotees, such a phenomenon could be explained as a coping strategy.[22] In other words, many schizophrenic patients look to religion as a means of managing their condition. Thus, in most cases their religiousness is not a product of a mental disorder but rather one coping facet among others.[23]

---

16 Cf. Peter L. Benson, "Religion and substance use," in *Religion and mental health*, ed. John F. Schumaker (New York: Oxford University Press, 1992): 211–220.

17 Cf. Dustin Pardini, Thomas G. Plante and Allen C. Sherman, "Strength of religious faith and its association with mental health outcomes among recovering alcoholics and addicts," *Journal of Substance Abuse Treatment 19* (2001): 347–354.

18 Cf. Sebastian Murken, "Das Konzept der Zwölf Schritte und der ‚Höheren Macht'. Zum Genesungsprogramm der Anonymen Alkoholiker," *Prävention* 31 (2008): 57–60.

19 Cf. Patricia L. Borman and David N. Dixon, "Spirituality and the 12 steps of substance abuse recovery," *Journal of Psychology and Theology 26* (1998): 287–291.

20 Cf. William P. Wilson, "Religion and psychoses," in *Handbook of religion and mental health*, ed. Harold G. Koenig (New York: Academic Press, 1998): 161–174.

21 Cf. Saheed Wahass and Gerry Kent, "Coping with auditory hallucinations: A cross-cultural comparison between Western (British) and non-Western (Saudi Arabian) patients," *Journal of Nervous and Mental Disease* 185 (1997): 664–668.

22 Cf. Joseph Z.T. Pieper, "Religious coping in highly religious inpatients," *Mental Health, Religion & Culture 7* (2004): 349–363; Leslie Tepper, Steven A. Rogers, Esther M. Coleman and H. Newton Malony, "The prevalence of religious coping among persons with persistent mental illness," *Psychiatric Services* 52 (2001): 660–665.

23 Cf. Sylvia Mohr, Christiane Gilliéron, Laurence Borras, Pierre-Yves Brandt and Philippe Huguelet, "The assessment of spirituality and religiousness in schizophrenia," *Journal of Nervous and Mental Disease* 195 (2007): 247–253.

2.5 Religiosity as Risk Factor

Since the end of the 1990s there has been a growing body of literature about possible negative aspects of religiosity which have been described as "religious struggle", "religious strain", or "religious conflict".[24] These terms cover in particular religious feelings of guilt, of fear of punishment, and of anger towards God or blaming God for personal suffering. The previous studies show that such negative aspects of religiosity are associated with lower mental and even physical health.[25] However, in many cases such feelings and attributions are rather temporary states during crises and conflicts when trying to cope with life events. Thus, they can alternatively be understood as passages during processes of personal growth.[26] This observation hints at the dynamic character of personal religiosity which undergoes lifelong changes and developments. Therefore, within health research religiosity should not be understood as a static but rather as a dynamic phenomenon.

2.6 Anxiety and Obsessive-Compulsive Disorders

Although results of studies are mixed, there seem to be rather negative correlations between intrinsic religiosity and anxiety or symptoms of anxiety.[27] Alternatively, consistent with the findings about religiosity as risk factor, there are also a substantial number of studies which indicate that religious beliefs

---

24 E.g. Julie J. Exline, "Religious and spiritual struggles," in *APA handbook of psychology, religion, and spirituality (Vol 1): Context, theory, and research*, eds. Kenneth I. Pargament, Julia J. Exline and James W. Jones (Washington, DC: American Psychological Association, 2013): 459–475; Julie J. Exline and Ephraim D. Rose, "Religious and spiritual struggles," in *Handbook of the psychology of religion and spirituality*, eds. Raymond F. Paloutzian and Crystal L. Park (New York: Guilford, 2005): 315–330; Julie J. Exline and Ephraim D. Rose, "Religious and spiritual struggles," in *Handbook of the psychology of religion and spirituality*. 2nd edition, eds. Raymond F. Paloutzian and Crystal L. Park (New York: Guilford, 2013): 380–398.

25 Cf. George Fitchett, Bruce D. Rybarczyk, Gail A. DeMarco and John J. Nicholas, "The role of religion in medical rehabilitation outcomes: A longitudinal study," *Rehabilitation Psychology 44* (1999): 1–22; Kenneth I. Pargament, Harold G. Koenig, Nalini Tarakeshwar and June Hahn, "Religious struggle as a predictor of mortality among medically ill elderly patients: A two-year longitudinal study," *Archives of Internal Medicine 161* (2001): 1881–1885.

26 Cf. Richard G. Tedeschi, Crystal L. Park and Lawrence G. Calhoun, eds., *Posttraumatic growth: Positive changes in the aftermath of crisis* (Mahwah, NJ: Erlbaum, 1998).

27 Cf. Kendler et al., "Clarifying the relationship between religiosity," 137–144.

can add to the formation and perpetuation of anxiety symptoms.[28] This seems to be true particularly for people whose religious upbringing has been very rigorous, for people who can be described as extrinsically religious or for people overstating religious concepts such as "sin". Although symptoms are often expressed through religious activities among highly religious obsessive-compulsive patients, obsessive-compulsive disorders are not more common among highly religious persons.[29]

3 Religiosity and Physical Health

Epidemiological studies show that religiosity has effects on mortality and thus seems to have an impact on physical health. The relevance of religiosity in coping with severe diseases has already been subject of empirical research. Here, however, the main interest is not in the relation between religiosity and physical health but in the existential and spiritual questions which arise when a severely ill person is confronted with her or his situation. It is the task of spiritual care to address these questions not only to palliative patients but also to people suffering from chronic illness. First results indicate the effectiveness of spiritual care concepts. The following paragraphs explicate these relations between religiosity and physical health.

3.1 Mortality

Epidemiological meta-analyses show that religiosity is associated with lower mortality rates in healthy populations so that higher religious people can be expected to live somewhat longer than the lower religious.[30] This epidemiological effect is not huge but quite robust. The association between religiosity and lower

---

28 Cf. Andrea K. Shreve-Neiger and Barry A. Edelstein, "Religion and anxiety: A critical review of the literature," *Clinical Psychology Review 24* (2004): 379–397.

29 Cf. Nancy Higgins, C. Alec Pollard and William T. Merkel, "Relationship between religion-related factors and obsessive compulsive disorder," *Current Psychology 11* (1992): 79–85; Frances J. Raphael, Shashi Rani, R. Bale and Lynne M. Drummond, "Religion, ethnicity and obsessive-compulsive disorder," *International Journal of Social Psychiatry 42* (1996): 38–44.

30 Cf. Yoishi Chida, Andrew Steptoe and Lynda H. Powell, "Religiosity/spirituality and mortality," *Psychotherapy and Psychosomatics 78* (2009): 81–90; Michael E. McCullough, William T. Hoyt, David B. Larson, Harold G. Koenig and Carl Thoresen, "Religious involvement and mortality: A meta-analytic review," *Health Psychology 19* (2000): 211–222.

mortality gets stronger in studies where religiosity has not been operationalized as private but as public practice. Thus the slightly higher longevity of religious people might be a consequence of benefits from social interactions and relationships,[31] and maybe also from positive emotions during services. Furthermore, the association between religiosity and lower mortality is stronger for women than men,[32] and is true in particular for mortality due to lifestyle related diseases.[33] It should also be noted that there is no statistical association between religiosity and lower mortality in diseased populations. If an illness has already occurred, religiosity does not affect progression or survival. Thus, religiosity seems to be more protective than curative.

3.2 Life-Threatening Diseases, in Particular Cancer

In surveys, patients suffering from life-threatening diseases often express their need for spiritual support and their wish to talk about religious issues, individual meaning and purpose, and about other existential topics.[34] It is well corroborated that religious beliefs can be a source of strength and hope for severely and terminally ill people. At the end of life, religiously committed persons seem to accept death better than nonreligious people.[35] Cancer is often seen as "prototype" of a life-threatening disease. Several reviews summarize the empirical results about the role of religiosity for coping with cancer.[36] Members of particular religious traditions have a lower risk of developing cancer. Conversely, like

---

31 Cf. Eran Shor and David Roelfs, "The longevity effects of religious and nonreligious participation: A meta-analysis and meta-regression," *Journal for the Scientific Study of Religion 52* (2013): 120–145.

32 Cf. Joana Maselko et al., "Religious service attendance and allostatic load among high-functioning elderly," *Psychosomatic Medicine 69* (2007): 464–472.

33 I.e. cardiovascular and respiratory diseases; cf. Chida et al., "Religiosity/spirituality and mortality," 81–90.

34 Cf. Paul S. Mueller, David J. Plevak and Teresa A. Rummans, "Religious involvement, spirituality, and medicine: Implications for clinical practice," *Mayo Clinic Proceedings 76* (2001): 1225–1235.

35 Cf. Dale A. Matthews et al., "Religious commitment and health status: A review of the research and implications for family medicine," *Archives of Family Medicine 7* (1998): 118–124.

36 Cf. Allen C. Sherman and Stephanie Simonton, "Spirituality and cancer," in *Spirit, science and health. How the spiritual mind fuels physical wellness*, eds. Thomas G. Plante and Carl E. Thoresen (Westport, CT: Praeger, 2007): 157–175; Michael Stefanek, Paige G. McDonald and Stephanie A. Hess, "Religion, spirituality and cancer: Current status and methodological challenges," *Psycho-Oncology 14* (2005): 450–463; Ingela C. Thuné-Boyle, Jan A. Stygall, Mohammed R. Keshtgar and Shanton Newman, "Do religious/spiritual coping strategies affect illness

other potentially fatal diseases, cancer is no exception when religiosity is introduced after diagnosis. Patients see no curative effect after acquiring religiousness as a coping mechanism. However, according to a meta-analysis by Heather S. Jim,[37] greater religiosity is at least associated with better patient-reported physical health in cancer patients.

3.3 Spiritual Care

Spiritual care deals in particular with the existential and religious/spiritual needs of patients suffering from life-threatening and chronic diseases; multiprofessional spiritual support could improve the subjective quality of life of the suffering.[38] The effectiveness of particular spiritual care interventions has not been studied intensively yet.[39] An American study revealed that patients with progressive cancer whose spiritual needs were not addressed satisfactorily expressed more depressive symptoms and less feelings of meaning and peace.[40] A randomized Japanese study showed that a week-long intervention including life review interviews could decrease the psychosocial burden and improve the impression of a "good death" among severely ill cancer patients.[41] Furthermore, there are correlative studies showing a positive association between the availability of spiritual care or prayer offers and the subjective quality of life of patients.[42]

---

adjustment in patients with cancer? A systematic review of the literature," *Social Science & Medicine 63* (2006): 151–164.

37 Cf. Heather S. Jim et al., "Religion, spirituality, and physical health in cancer patients: A meta-analysis," *Cancer 121* (2015): 3760–3768.

38 Cf. Eckhard Frick, "Spiritual Care in der Humanmedizin: Profilierung und Vernetzung," in *Gesundheit – Religion – Spiritualität. Konzepte, Befunde und Erklärungsansätze*, eds. Constantin Klein, Hendrik Berth and Friedrich Balck (Weinheim: Juventa, 2011): 407–420.

39 Cf. Marjolein Gysels and Irene J. Higginson, *Improving supportive and palliative care for adults with cancer. Research evidence* (London: National Institute for Clinical Excellence, 2004); Margret Holloway, Sue Adamson, Wilf McSherry and John Swinton, *Spiritual care at the end of life: A systematic review of the literature* (Hull: University of Hull, Department of Health, 2011); Naomi Kalish, "Evidence-based spiritual care: A literature review," *Current Opinion in Supportive and Palliative Care 6* (2012): 242–246.

40 Cf. Michelle J. Pearce et al., "Unmet spiritual care needs impact emotional and spiritual well-being," *Supportive Care in Cancer 20* (2012): 2269–2276.

41 Cf. Michiyo Ando, Tatsuya Morita, Tatsuo Akechi and Takuya Okamoto, "Efficacy of short-term life-review interviews on the spiritual well-being of terminal ill cancer patients," *Journal of Pain and Symptom Management 39* (2010): 993–1002.

42 Cf. Naomi Kalish, "Evidence-based spiritual care: A literature review," *Current Opinion in Supportive and Palliative Care 6* (2012): 242–246.

4 Possible Pathways from Religiosity to Health

What are the pathways in which religiosity can affect mental and physical health positively or negatively; which mediators can be detected between both constructs? Possible explanations can be integrated into a heuristic framework,[43] which is aligned to the basic ideas of the diathesis-stress model[44] and the transactional model of stress and coping[45] as Figure 1 illustrates.

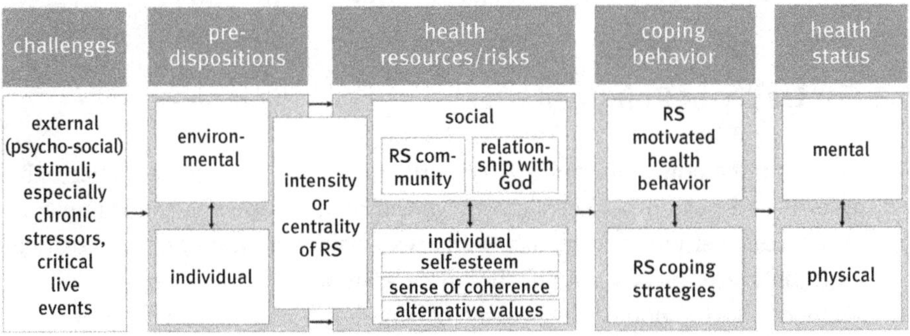

Figure 1: Heuristic Framework for the Illustration of Possible Pathways from Religiosity to Health*. *Cf. Klein and Albani, „Die Bedeutung von Religion für die psychische Befindlichkeit," 7–58; Klein and Albani, „Religiosität und psychische Gesundheit," 215–245; Zwingmann and Klein, "Deutschsprachige Fragebogenskalen zur Messung von Religiosität/Spiritualität," 7–21.

According to the framework in Figure 1, an individual's mental and partially physical *health status* is the result of reactions to external *stimuli and challenges*, in particular daily hassles, chronic stressors, or critical life events. The

43 Cf. Constantin Klein and Cornelia Albani, "Die Bedeutung von Religion für die psychische Befindlichkeit: Mögliche Erklärungsansätze und allgemeines Wirkmodell," *Zeitschrift für Nachwuchswissenschaftler* 3 (2011): 7–58; Constantin Klein and Cornelia Albani, "Religiosität und psychische Gesundheit – empirische Befunde und Erklärungsansätze," in *Gesundheit – Religion – Spiritualität. Konzepte, Befunde und Erklärungsansätze*, eds. Constantin Klein, Hendrik Berth and Friedrich Balck (Weinheim: Juventa, 2011): 215–245; Christian Zwingmann and Constantin Klein, „Deutschsprachige Fragebogenskalen zur Messung von Religiosität/Spiritualität: Stellenwert, Klassifikation und Auswahlkriterien," *Spiritual Care* 1(3) (2012): 7–21.

44 Cf. Rick E. Ingram and Joseph M. Price, *Vulnerability to psychopathology. Risk across the lifespan* (New York: Guilford, 2001); Marvin Zuckerman, *Vulnerability to psychopathology. A biosocial model* (Washington, DC: American Psychological Association, 1999).

45 Cf. Folkman, "Positive psychological states," 1207–1221; Lazarus and Folkman, *Stress, appraisal, and coping*.

reactions consist of several interacting factors: Among them are at first individual *predispositions*, which are either hereditary or socialized by the environment. Furthermore, social and individual *health resources and risk factors*, which generally determine how the individual reacts to challenges can contribute to health outcomes. The last factors in the model, which are most closely related to the health status are preventive *health-related behavior* (e.g., lifestyle factors such as moderate substance consumption or sobriety) and *coping strategies* which are used to cope with the prevailing challenges. Religiosity can play a positive or negative role for several factors within the framework.

4.1 Centrality of Religiosity

Due to the huge amount of findings about the impact of intrinsic religiosity, the centrality of religiosity has been given a prominent position in the framework between predispositions and health resources – as the centrality of religiosity is related to both groups of variables. It can be assumed that the effects of all further elements in the model will become stronger and more distinguished if the centrality of religiosity is expressed on a high level.[46] A meta-analysis undertaken by Hackney and Sanders[47] over 34 studies shows impressively that measures of intrinsic religiosity and personal devotion correlate stronger with health indicators than measures of institutionalized or ideological religiosity.

4.2 Social Support of the Religious Community

Social support is a well-known important protective factor of health. It is plausible that involvement in the social network of a religious community can have salutary effects through concrete support. Social networks can help with illness and critical life events through the camaraderie of trustful relationships and/or community. There is empirical evidence from the US that religious people, in particular the elderly, have bigger and more stable social networks and receive more social support.[48] Longitudinal studies show that persons who attend

46 Cf. Huber, *Zentralität und Inhalt.*

47 Cf. Charles H. Hackney and Glenn S. Sanders, "Religiosity and mental health: A meta-analysis of recent studies," *Journal for the Scientific Study of Religion 42* (2003): 43–55.

48 Cf. Koenig et al., Handbook of religion and health; Douglas Oman and Dwayne Reed, "Religion and mortality among the community-dwelling elderly," *American Journal of Public Health 88* (1998): 1469–1475.

church on a regular basis are at a lower risk to be socially isolated.[49] But in extreme cases social support provided by religious communities can also become negative. A common example of negative social support is social control where members of a religious community are isolated due to nonobservance to group rules or if a religious group culturally and socially segregates itself from the larger society. Basically groups with aggressive attempts to control adherent's behavior and relationships are detrimental to the individuals.[50]

4.3 Relationship with God and Self-Esteem

The relationship with God (and other transcendent entities with potential otherworldly reciprocity) can be understood as a particular type of attachment and can in the best case stimulate feelings of ultimate trust and being accepted which might lead to positive salutary self-esteem.[51] In the worst case, however, the relationship with God can generate negative feelings like fear of temptation, sin, and divine punishment and can possibly be detrimental to self-esteem and mental health.[52]

4.4 Sense of Coherence

Sense of coherence as described by Antonovsky[53] is expected to be an important protective factor, too. The concept encompasses an orientation experiencing the world to be comprehensive, manageable, and meaningful. Religious traditions provide extensive explanations and cognitive schemes which can be useful for a

---

49 Cf. William J. Strawbridge, Sarah J. Shema, Richard D. Cohen and George A. Kaplan, "Religious attendance increases survival by improving and maintaining good health practices, mental health, and stable marriages," *Annals of Behavioral Medicine 23* (2001): 68–74.

50 Cf. Heinz Streib et al., *Deconversion. Qualitative and quantitative results from cross-cultural research in Germany and the United States of America* (Göttingen: Vandenhoeck & Ruprecht, 2009).

51 Cf. Lee A. Kirkpatrick, *Attachment, evolution, and the psychology of religion* (New York: Guilford, 2004).

52 Cf. Julie J. Exline, Crystal L. Park, Joshua M. Smyth and Michael P. Carey, "Anger toward God: Social-cognitive predictors, prevalence, and links with adjustment to bereavement and cancer," *Journal of Personality and Social Psychology 100* (2011): 129–148; Sebastian Murken, *Gottesbeziehung und psychische Gesundheit. Die Entwicklung eines Modells und seine empirische Überprüfung* (Münster: Waxmann, 1998).

53 Cf. Aaron Antonovsky, "The structure and properties of the Sense of Coherence Scale," *Social Science & Medicine 36* (1993): 725–733.

meaningful interpretation of the complex challenges and demands of life.[54] This can be helpful in particular cases of loss and suffering.[55] But religious interpretations might potentially become dangerous for one's mental health if they are understood too rigidly, for instance if they include contents which are experienced as fear of rejection by God or as divine punishment.[56] In social perspective, rigid religious beliefs might become critical when their message becomes physically dangerous to others such as repression of freedoms of minorities or when they cause disruption within democracy.

4.5 Alternative Values and Religiously Motivated Health Behavior

Religious norms provide health-related and alternative social rules of behavior. It is possible that religious rules for nutrition, hygiene, and sexuality affect health directly and indirectly by reducing self-damaging behavior and advocating preventive attitudes. Studies on smaller denominations with strict norms such as Latter-day Saints or Seventh Day Adventists illustrate that religious communities can effectively support a healthy lifestyle.[57] But religiosity seems also to be associated with less smoking, drinking of alcohol, drug abuse, and more use of preventive activities in less strict denominations among adults and adolescents.[58] Here,

---

54 Cf. Kenneth E. Vail et al., "Terror management analysis of the psychological functions of religion," *Personality and Social Psychology Review 14* (2010): 84–94.

55 Cf. Daniel McIntosh, "Religion as a schema, with implications for the relation between religion and coping," *International Journal for the Psychology of Religion 5* (1995): 1–16; Hansjörg Znoj, Christoph Morgenthaler and Christian Zwingmann, "Mehr als nur Bewältigen? Religiosität, Stressreaktionen und Coping bei elterlicher Depressivität nach dem Verlust eines Kindes," in *Religiosität: Messverfahren und Studien zu Gesundheit und Lebensqualität. Neue Beiträge zur Religionspsychologie*, eds. Christian Zwingmann and Helfried Moosbrugger (Münster: Waxmann, 2004): 277–297.

56 Cf. Julie J. Exline, Crystal L. Park, Joshua M. Smyth and Michael P. Carey, "Anger toward God: Social-cognitive predictors, prevalence, and links with adjustment to bereavement and cancer," *Journal of Personality and Social Psychology 100* (2011): 129–148.

57 Cf. R.L. Phillips and D.A. Snowdon, "Association of meat and coffee use with cancers of the large bowel, breast, and prostate among Seventh-Day Adventists: Preliminary results," *Cancer Research 43* (5 Suppl.) (1983): 2403–2408; Henry Troyer, "Review of cancer among 4 religious sects: Evidence that life-styles are distinctive sets of risk factors," *Social Science & Medicine* 26 (1988): 1007–1017.

58 Cf. Sian Cotton, Daniel H. Grossoehme and Joel Tsevat, "Religion/spirituality and health in adolescents," in *Spirit, science and health. How the spiritual mind fuels physical wellness*, eds. Thomas G. Plante and Carl E. Thoresen (Westport, CT: Praeger, 2007): 143–156; Andreas Hoff

the effect of religiosity seems to be rather indirect as a result of the imparting of values like appreciation of the body, valuing family life, or avoidance of excesses.[59] Religious norms further emphasize alternative values like humility, abstinence, and charity instead of power, luxury, and self-enhancement. They can thus encourage virtues like forgiveness,[60] and gratitude,[61] and contribute to a reduction of social distress. Although the implications of religious rules for health are typically positive, the opposite is possible. In some smaller denominations, for instance, some medical treatments are rejected which can sometimes result in avoidable cases of death.[62]

4.6 Religious Coping

Religiosity can play an important role in the effective coping with stress and diseases. Therefore, researchers such as Folkman have explicitly integrated several *meaning-based coping strategies* including spiritual coping into the transactional stress-coping model of Lazarus and Folkman.[63] According to this modified model, meaning-based coping is used to perpetuate coping activities when other coping strategies did not succeed. Religious coping has been studied extensively during the last 25 years.[64] The current state of research can be

et al., "Religion and reduced cancer risk – What is the explanation? A review," *European Journal of Cancer Care 17* (2008): 2573–2579; Koenig et al., Handbook of religion and health; Ha Koenig et al., Handbook of religion and health. 2nd edition. Yonker et al., "The relationship between spirituality and religiosity," 299–314.

59 Cf. Bernhard Grom, "Gesundheit und ‚Glaubensfaktor'. Religiosität als Komplementärmedizin?," *Stimmen der Zeit 216* (1998): 413–424.

60 Cf. Michael E. McCullough, Kenneth I. Pargament and Carl E. Thoresen, eds., *Forgiveness. Theory, research, and practice* (New York: Guilford, 2000).

61 Cf. Michael E. McCullough, Robert A. Emmons and Jo-Ann Tsang, "The grateful disposition: A conceptual and empirical topography," *Journal of Personality and Social Psychology 82* (2002): 112–127.

62 Cf. Seth M. Asser and Rita Swan, "Child fatalities from religion-motivated medical neglect," *Pediatrics 101* (1998): 625–629.

63 Cf. Susan Folkman, "Positive psychological states and coping with severe stress," *Social Science & Medicine 45* (1997): 1207–1221; Richard S. Lazarus and Susan Folkman, *Stress, appraisal, and coping* (New York: Springer, 1984).

64 Cf. Gene G. Ano and Erin B. Vasconcelles, "Religious coping and psychosocial adjustment to stress: A meta-analysis," *Journal of Clinical Psychology 61* (2005): 1–20; Kenneth I. Pargament, *The psychology of religion and coping. Theory, research, practice* (New York: Guilford, 1997); Kenneth I. Pargament, *Spiritually integrated psychotherapy: Understanding and addressing the sacred* (New York: Guilford, 2007); Terry Lynn Gall and Manal Guirguis-Younger, "Religious and

subsumed as follows: 1. Religious coping is preferred in comparison to nonreligious coping in particular in situations of severe burden and loss, i.e. in situations when the limits and not the potentials of human existence matter. 2. Although the findings are not completely homogenous, religious coping seems not to be functionally redundant to nonreligious coping. There are indeed moderate associations between religious and nonreligious coping strategies. However, religious coping predicts health outcomes above and beyond the contribution of nonreligious coping. 3. Religiosity can affect coping to the positive as well as to the negative. According to existing research, an individual may find particularly the following positive strategies in religiousness: One may seek relief through a focus on religiosity. They may look for a stronger relationship with God. The individual may be searching for comfort and reassurance through God's love and care. They may be seeking control through a partnership with God in problem-solving. They might find reappraisal of the stressor as challenge or strengthening by God. Finally they may be looking to religion for help in shifting from anger, hurt, and fear. It has been discovered that negative coping strategies incur discontent with the relationship with God, discontent with the relationship with clergy or members of the religious community, questioning the power of God, reappraisal of the stressor as God's punishment, and reappraisal of the stressor as an act of the devil. 4. Positive religious coping is much more common and contributes to a better coping outcome. Negative religious coping is rather seldom but affects the coping process strongly for the worse. 5. Positive and negative coping can be used simultaneously.

---

spiritual coping: Current theory and research," in *APA handbook of psychology, religion, and spirituality (Vol 1): Context, theory, and research*, eds. Kenneth I. Pargament, Julie J. Exline and James W. Jones (Washington, DC: American Psychological Association 2013): 349–364; Kenneth I. Pargament, Gene G. Ano and Amy B. Wachholtz, "The religious dimensions of coping: Advances in theory, research, and practice," in *Handbook of the psychology of religion and spirituality*, eds. Raymond F. Paloutzian and Crystal L. Park (New York: Guilford, 2005): 479–495; Kenneth I. Pargament, Melissa D. Falb, Gene G. Ano and Amy B. Wachholtz, "The religious dimension of coping: Advances in theory, research, and practice," in *Handbook of the psychology of religion and spirituality*. 2nd edition, eds. Raymond F. Paloutzian and Crystal L. Park (New York: Guilford, 2013): 560–580.

5 Evidence from a Secular Context: Findings from the German-Speaking Countries

95 % of US Americans confirm that they believe in God – a rate which has been almost constant since 1944 and much higher than in the German-speaking countries (Switzerland: 59 %, West Germany: 53 %, Austria: 47 %, East Germany: 13 %).[65] Additionally, there is an ongoing decrease of religious affiliation within the German-speaking countries. Similar differences can also be found for other indicators of individual religiosity.[66] Furthermore, the social impact of religious practice is much higher in the US than in Europe. The American model, of course, is an open market of potential religious communities for anyone seeking to belong. Moreover, many of these communities include evangelical and pentecostal movements where proselytization and religious conversion are commonplace. Affiliation and networking produces the potential for social capital from members helping each other to prayer.[67] Finally, religious beliefs and public religious rhetoric are important parts of political life in the US.[68]

Due to the immense cultural differences, research results about religiosity and health from the American context cannot easily be transferred to the more secularized German-speaking countries. A recent meta-analysis including 67 studies conducted in Germany, Austria, and German-speaking Switzerland indicates that greater religiosity is only very weakly albeit significantly associated with better mental health in the German-speaking area.[69] The results are not or only slightly moderated by study and sociodemographic characteristics. However, the results are substantially moderated by the type of religiosity measure used in the studies: "Maladaptive dealing with religion and God" correlates substantially negatively with mental health, whereas all other measures of

65 Cf. Stefan Huber, "Religiosität in Deutschland, Österreich und der Schweiz," in *Gesundheit – Religion – Spiritualität. Konzepte, Befunde und Erklärungsansätze*, eds. Constantin Klein, Hendrik Berth and Friedrich Balck (Weinheim: Juventa, 2011): 172.

66 Cf. Bertelsmann Stiftung, ed., *Religionsmonitor 2008* (Gütersloh: Bertelsmann Stiftung, 2009).

67 Cf. Rodney Stark and Roger Finke, *Acts of faith: Explaining the human side of religion* (Berkeley, CA: University of California Press, 2000).

68 Cf. Stiftung, *Religionsmonitor 2008*.

69 Cf. Bastian Hodapp, *Religiosität/Spiritualität und psychische Gesundheit – eine Metaanalyse über Studien aus dem deutschsprachigen Raum* (Hamburg: Kovač, 2017); Bastian Hodapp and Christian Zwingmann, "Religiosity/Spirituality and mental health: a meta-analysis of studies from the German-speaking area," *Journal of Religion and Health* 58 (2019): 1970–1998; Christian Zwingmann and Bastian Hodapp, "Religiosität/Spiritualität und psychische Gesundheit: Zentrale Ergebnisse einer Metaanalyse über Studien aus dem deutschsprachigen Raum," *Spiritual Care* 7 (2018): 69–80.

religiosity predominantly exhibit small positive associations. In comparison to US-American meta-analyses, the average effect size based on studies from the German-speaking area is lower. Furthermore, the associations between negative types of religiosity and lower mental health are particularly strong. For instance, it was reported that worse mental health was related to a negative relationship with God,[70] and lower subjective well-being, more anxiety and depression was related to negative religious coping,[71] in particular when the centrality of religiosity is on a high level.[72]

6 Summary and Conclusions

It can be recapitulated from the overview that – at least in the US – an intrinsic and personally relevant religiosity is associated with better mental and physical health. However, the correlations are often rather low and the direction of statistical effects mostly remains unclear. There are distinct possible pathways from religiosity to health which do not exclude each other and which have been investigated with differing intensity. Notwithstanding these limitations, the results still show that it makes sense to use religious resources within medical and therapeutic treatment.[73] However, an intrinsic religiosity can only be "used" if it already exists, but can never be "prescribed". Moreover, the integration of religiosity into medical history and therapy is important, because it is possible – although seldom – that religiosity can affect health to the worse, such as those cases with feelings of anxiety and guilt. It can be helpful then to strengthen positive religious coping strategies.

70 Cf. Murken, *Gottesbeziehung und psychische Gesundheit.*

71 Cf. Urs Winter et al., "The psychological outcome of religious coping with stressful life events in a Swiss sample of church attendees," *Psychotherapy and Psychosomatics* 78 (2009): 240–244.

72 Cf. Christian Zwingmann, Claudia Müller, Jürgen Körber and Sebastian Murken, "Religious commitment, religious coping and anxiety: A study in German patients with breast cancer," *European Journal of Cancer Care 17* (2008): 361–370.

73 Cf. Eckhard Frick and Traugott Roser, eds., *Spiritualität und Medizin. Gemeinsame Sorge für den kranken Menschen* (Stuttgart: Kohlhammer, 2011); Edward P. Shafranske, ed., *Religion and the clinical practice of psychology* (Washington, DC: American Psychological Association, 1996); Edward P. Shafranske, "The psychology of religion in clinical and counseling psychology," in *Handbook of the psychology of religion and spirituality*, eds. Raymond F. Paloutzian and Crystal L. Park (New York: Guilford, 2005): 496–514.

Findings about the relation between religiosity and health from the US cannot be generalized by implication. There are desiderata in particular with respect to non-Christian religions and secularized countries; intercultural comparisons have been claimed stronger only recently. In comparison to US-American meta-analytic results, a recent meta-analysis from the German language area revealed a very small average association between religiosity and mental health and, furthermore, particular strong relationships between negative types of religiosity and lower mental health. The cultural context thus seems to be of high relevance for the pattern of how religiosity and health are intertwined.[74]

---

74 Cf. Heinz Streib and Constantin Klein, "Atheists, agnostics, and apostates," in *APA handbook of psychology, religion, and spirituality (Vol 1): Context, theory, and research*, eds. Kenneth I. Pargament, Julie J. Exline and James W. Jones (Washington, DC: American Psychological Association, 2013): 713–728.

Annette Haußmann

Depression and Spirituality/Religion

An Ambivalent Relationship

1 Introduction

Depression is one of the most common mental diseases and is influenced by various factors, including religion and spirituality which are largely found to have a positive impact on depression[1]. But religion and spirituality can also influence a depressive mood by increasing depressive symptoms. This intertwined relationship between religion and depression can best be understood as embedded in a complex model of religious coping. When religious people fall ill, they continue to be religious beings – with specific convictions and beliefs, religious behavior and spiritual needs which play an important part in their daily lives. Also, depression can change the religiousness of a person. Attending a Sunday service becomes as difficult as any other social activity because of the lack of energy and hopelessness. A person suffering from concentration difficulties may no longer remember the Lord's Prayer and a personal prayer seems to be pointless. And finally, the access to feelings like gratitude, forgiveness or trust in God can become impossible because of the illness. To some, during such times of internal darkness, God seems distant, they may even question His existence, and everything that gave meaning to their life appears to fade away. Some people who are religious suffer from guilt caused by the change in their psychic system. It is therefore important to see these changes in the context of the illness and not primarily as a crisis of faith caused by a faith that is too weak. It can be an existential burdening experience when the usual confidence in faith disappears as well. Apart from all the other aspects in life that are affected by depression, the loss of faith weighs heavily and can be described as an infinite loneliness, resembling death or hell for highly religious people. Here, pastoral care can be helpful and supportive to meet the specific spiritual needs during the illness in addition to specialized psychotherapeutic treatment.

1 The following article is based on the project "Depression and Church Congregations" and on the resulting article by Birgit Weyel and Annette Haußmann, "Spiritualität und Depressivität," in *Menschen mit Depression. Orientierungen und Impulse für die Praxis in Kirchengemeinden*, eds. Birgit Weyel and Beate Jakob (Gütersloh: Gütersloher Verlagshaus, 2014): 19–26.

https://doi.org/10.1515/9783110674217-004

The term "depression" is normally used to name a mental disorder. There are a variety of affective disorders which fall into this category – ranging from a major depressive episode, dysthymia[2], cyclothymia[3] to bipolar disorder[4]. On the other hand, depression can also name a state with depressive mood – from temporary discontentment, sadness, burden to a negative emotional state and lack of motivation or the loss of energy.[5] I will use the term "depression" in this article to name the whole spectrum of depressive symptoms and moods. Both, a mild displeasure or a manifest depressive episode can have an impact on the individual's religious system that contains beliefs, practices and emotions. It furthermore also influences the individual's social environment and thus, e.g. can impair the engagement in a religious community or close social relationships. Therefore, it seems reasonable to talk about a holistic depressive influence on every human sphere.

As the results of our empirical study have shown on a qualitative level, during a depressive episode, people experience a variety of phenomena that also include the spiritual and religious dimension.[6] It can range from the sudden feeling of being forgotten by God, not being able to pray anymore, but also positively experiencing closeness to God during a walk through the woods.[7] These results will be put in the context of current research in the field of psychology of religion and practical theology. The definition of religion and/or spirituality is a challenging task: Whereas some scholars clearly distinguish both terms,[8]

2 Dysthymia (F34.1) is a chronic depressive state in which patients do not fulfil the full criteria of a major depression but show several depressive symptoms constantly over time.

3 Cyclothymia (F34.0) also is a chronic depressive state that leads to swaying mood passages, but at no time fulfils the criteria of a major depression episode.

4 Patients with a bipolar affective disorder are switching between depressive episodes and episodes of mania or hypomania.

5 Cf. Harold G. Koenig, Dana E. King and Verna B. Carson, *Handbook of religion and health*, 2. Edition (Oxford: Oxford University Press, 2012): 145–173.

6 Cf. chapter II.3 in this volume: Beate Jakob, *Is faith a Source of Strength? Do Congregations offer Support? A Qualitative Study with People Affected by Mental Disorders and Their Relatives.*

7 These examples are taken from the original interviews, conducted by Stefanie Koch, published in Stefanie Koch, "Wie können Kirchengemeinden depressiv kranke Menschen und ihre Angehörigen unterstützen? Interviews mit ausgewählten Personengruppen," in *Menschen mit Depression: Orientierungen und Impulse für die Praxis in Kirchengemeinden*, eds. Birgit Weyel, Beate Jakob and Stefanie Koch (Gütersloh: Gütersloher Verlagshaus, 2014): 53–97.

8 Mostly, spirituality is considered the broader construct, including non-institutionalized, secularized forms of beliefs and practices, whereas religion on the other hand is often identified with an institutionalized view, like a certain denomination or world religion. For an integrative definition of religion and spirituality cf. e.g. Brian J. Zinnbauer and Kenneth I. Pargament, "Religiousness and spirituality," in *Handbook of the Psychology of Religion and Spirituality*,

I will use the terms 'religion' and 'spirituality' synonymously, assuming that every individual has certain thoughts and needs about religion and spirituality, including worldviews, meaning making, and transcendence. I will also refer to the multidimensionality of religion and spirituality, which includes cognition, emotion, behavior, motivation, and the social sphere.[9] Acknowledging that various cultural and denominational differences exist, I will primarily concentrate on studies from a monotheistic Christian background; since research is international, results from various countries, but mostly from the US will be presented.

In this article, I will describe current empirical studies (2), followed by theoretical frameworks, as suggested by Kenneth Pargament and Julie Exline to explain the relation between depression and religion and further variables which supposedly influence this relationship (3). Then, I will focus on phenomena that are often experienced by depressed individuals and also observed in clinical studies (4). Following this, I will describe how religion can also have a preventive or alleviating effect on depressive symptoms (5). Finally, some ideas of how to deal with depression and religion will be given from a psychotherapeutic and pastoral care position (6).

2 Overview of Empirical Results

Empirical research in the field of depression and religion or spirituality has increased significantly over the last 20 years. Whereas in 1998 there were only roughly 100 studies,[10] Smith et al. included 147 studies in 2003[11] and then 445

eds. Raymond F. Paloutzian and Crystal L. Park (Princeton/New York: Guilford Press, 2005): 21–42. Interestingly, some scholars also point out the different influence of spirituality versus religiosity on depression. Cf. Jeffrey R. Vittengl, "A Lonely Search? Risk for Depression: When Spirituality Exceeds Religiosity," *The Journal of Nervous and Mental Disease 206, Issue 5* (2018): 386–389.

9 This multidimensional approach is wide spread in current psychology of religion, cf. e.g. Kenneth I. Pargament, Annette Mahoney, Julie J. Exline., James W. Jones and Edward P. Shafranske, "Envisioning an integrative paradigm for the psychology of religion and spirituality," in *APA Handbook of Psychology, Religion, and Spirituality: Vol. 1: Context, Theory, and Research*, ed. Kenneth I. Pargament (Washington D.C: American Psychological Association, 2013): 3–19.

10 Cf. Gary J. Kennedy, "Religion and Depression," in *Handbook of Religion and mental health*, ed. Harold G. Koenig (San Diego: Academic Press, 1998): 130–145.

11 Cf. Timothy B. Smith, Michael E. McCullough and Justin Poll, "Religiousness and depression: Evidence for a main effect and the moderating influence of stressful life events," *Psychological Bulletin* 129(4) (2003): 614–636.

quantitative studies were presented in the summary of Koenig et al. in 2012.[12] Considering that there are also theological, sociological and qualitative studies relating to this topic, the number of studies has increased immensely in a short period of time. However, the results of the quantitative – mostly cross-sectional – studies indicate that there are mostly positive relationships between religion and depression: two-thirds of the studies show that higher relevance of religion is associated with less depression or can lead to faster recovery from depressive episodes. On the other hand, 22% of the relevant studies also show no association between the two variables, and another 6% reveal a negative relationship in which higher religiosity is associated with greater depression.[13] Older reviews also showed robust positive effects of religion on depression.[14] The study of Bjørkløf et al. also found a stronger effect on depression reduction in individuals who express a higher importance of religion.[15] These reviews point to the complexity of the relationship between religion and depression and also focus on a central problem: the definition and measurement can be diverse and the results strongly depend on the operationalization of religion and spirituality. Because religion and spirituality are both complex constructs with elements of cognition, emotion, social implications, we can assume that in research we have to deal with a multidimensional construct that needs various measurements to discover multiple levels of influence on mental health.[16] Therefore, quantitative results are just the first step to understanding the intertwined relationship of both variables. Growing research has focused on the 'dark side' of religion and spirituality in the last years and point to a possible negative relationship between depression and religion depending on the content of religious and spiritual beliefs and practices.[17] Thus, we can assume that the connection between religion and depression is highly ambivalent. Furthermore, it is important to notice that it is more appropriate to talk about correlation and association, whereas causality can only

---

12 Cf. Koenig et al., *Handbook of religion and health*, 145–173.

13 Cf. Koenig et al., *Handbook of religion and health*, 145–173.

14 Cf. Peter H. Ness and David B. Larson, "Religion, Senescence, and Mental Health," *American Journal of Geriatric Psychiatry* 10(4) (2002): 386–397.

15 Cf. Guro H. Bjørkløf, Knut Engedal, Geir Selbæk, Siren E. Kouwenhoven and Anne-Sofie Helvik, "Coping and depression in old age: A literature review," *Dementia and geriatric cognitive disorders* 35 (2013): 3–4 and 121–154.

16 Latest research also points out that, considering longitudinal data, spirituality and religion are having different effects on different dimensions. Cf. Clayton H. McClintock et al., "Multidimensional understanding of religiosity/spirituality: relationship to major depression and familial risk," *Psychological medicine* (2018): 1–10.

17 Cf. Christian Zwingmann, Constantin Klein and Florian Jeserich (eds.), Religiosität: Die dunkle Seite: Beiträge zur empirischen Religionsforschung (Münster/New York: Waxmann, 2017).

be addressed with longitudinal research. Some studies have focused on long-term implications of religious belief on depression. Wink et al. found that, after statistically excluding social support as an influencing factor, religiosity had a positive influence on health, resulting in less depression in the course of a 5 year study.[18] The study of Miller et al. points again to the relevance of religion in the individual's orienting system indicating that stronger belief has more impact on depressive symptoms.[19]

German reviews mostly summarize Anglo-American results,[20] but it is important to notice the cultural differences that also influence the relationship between depression and religion. Anette Dörr and Urs Winter have successfully shown the relationship between depression and religion, mostly reporting that positive religious coping supports whereas negative religious coping increases depression.[21] A recent meta-analysis of 67 German studies from Zwingmann and Hodapp shows smaller overall effects for a German context between religion and health than in studies from the US context. Stronger effects are observed for 'negative dealing with God or religion' that influence health negatively, whereas other variables

18 Cf. Paul Wink, Michaela Dollin and Britta Larsen, "Religion as Moderator of the Depression-Health Connection: Findings from a Longitudinal Study," *Research on Aging* 27(2) (2005): 197–220. The authors measured religiosity as institutionalized religion (e.g. belief in God, an afterlife, church attendance, prayer) separately from non-institutionalized spirituality (e.g. meditation, belief in a higher power or God) and also found a stronger effect for institutionalized religiosity.

19 Cf. Lisa Miller, Priva Wickramaratne, Marc J. Gameroff, Mia Sage, Craig E. Tenke and Myrna M. Weissman, "Religiosity and major depression in adults at high risk: A ten-year prospective study," *The American Journal of Psychiatry* 169(1) (2012): 89–94.

20 Cf. Aarjan W. Braam, "Religion und Depression," in *Gesundheit – Religion – Spiritualität: Konzepte, Befunde und Erklärungsansätze*, eds. Constantin Klein, Hendrik Berth and Friedrich Balck (Weinheim: Beltz Juventa, 2011): 273–290; Samuel Pfeifer, "Seelenfinsternis und dunkle Nacht der Seele – Depression und Spiritualität," in *Psychotherapie und Spiritualität: Mit existenziellen Konflikten und Transzendenzfragen professionell umgehen*, eds. Michael Utsch, Raphael M. Bonelli and Samuel Pfeifer (Berlin/Heidelberg: Springer, 2014): 121–132 and Friedel M. Reischies, "Religiös-spirituelle Dimension bei psychischen Krankheiten – Depression: Positive und negative Auswirkungen religiösen Erlebens," *Spiritual Care* 6(1) (2017): 31–35.

21 Cf. Anette Dörr, *Religiosität und Depression: Eine empirisch-psychologische Untersuchung* (Weinheim: Deutscher Studien-Verlag, 1987); Anette Dörr, "Religiöses Coping als Ressource bei der Bewältigung von Life Events," in *Religiosität: Messverfahren und Studien zu Gesundheit und Lebensbewältigung. Neue Beiträge zur Religionspsychologie*, eds. Christian Zwingmann and Helfried Moosbrugger (Münster: Waxmann, 2004): 261–276 and Urs Christian Winter, *"Der Liebe Gott hat es so gewollt": die Rolle der Religiosität bei der Bewältigung kritischer Lebensereignisse sowie Impulse für eine pastorale Krisenintervention – eine pastoralpsychologische Studie* (Dissertation) (Fribourg: 2005).

like positive coping behavior, spirituality, and centrality of religion or an intrinsic religiosity had only a small but positive influence on health.[22] Also, a variety of experiences from pastoral care professionals indicate that depression is associated with religious or spiritual struggles and darkened God- and self-images.[23]

3 Theoretical Framework Explaining the Relationship between Depression and Religion

From what we know today, depression always roots in genetic factors and vulnerabilities and is best understood in process-oriented stress models that include factors that facilitate depressions, assuming that there are always multiple factors interacting resulting in depressive symptoms.[24] However, since the causes and results of depression are interrelated, it is reasonable to mention stressors, personal factors, illness-maintaining factors (cf. 4.), and resourceful factors that buffer or protect from depression (cf. 5.).[25] If religion is added to a model of understanding depression, two closely related theoretical frameworks can be mentioned.

3.1 Religious Coping Theory

Kenneth I. Pargament developed the theory of religious coping.[26] On the basis of a religious orienting system, which is rooted in religious education, socialization,

22 Cf. Christian Zwingmann and Bastian Hodapp, "Religiosität/Spiritualität und psychische Gesundheit: Zentrale Ergebnisse einer Metaanalyse über Studien aus dem deutschsprachigen Raum," *Spiritual Care* 7(1) (2017): 69–80.

23 Those observations are merely qualitative results from pastoral care interaction, cf. e.g. Kevin Culligan, "Vom Umgang mit der Dunkelheit in der geistlichen Begleitung," in *'Dunkle Nacht' und Depression: Geistliche und psychische Krisen verstehen und unterscheiden*, eds. Regina Bäumer and Michael Plattig (Ostfildern: Grünewald, 2008): 58–74.

24 Cf. Eva-Lotta Brakemeier, Claus Normann and Mathias Berger, "Ätiopathogenese der unipolaren Depression," Bundesgesundheitsblatt-Gesundheitsforschung-Gesundheitsschutz 51(4) (2008): 379–391.

25 Braam has systematized those aspects of biographical factors, development, symptoms, and process that interact with the different dimensions of religion into a matrix. Cf. Braam, "Religion und Depression," 273–290.

26 Cf. Kenneth I. Pargament, *The Psychology of Religion and Coping: Theory, research, practice* (New York: Guilford Press, 1997).

and personal experience, the individual develops values, practices, cognitions and emotions about God, the world, and the self. The more important religion and spirituality are in someone's life, the more influential religion is on mental health.[27] In times of stress, people react with a specific religious coping style, with various outcomes on mental health depending on the content of the religious orienting system.[28] Therefore, religion can either be primarily a protective factor and a resource, resulting in lower distress, or it can have harmful effects on mental health by e.g. intensifying current feelings like hopelessness, cognitive rumination or lower self-esteem. These various effects on coping can only be discovered and described on the basis of the individual's biography and development. Religious coping is a process that has different stages and leads through times of spiritual struggles by using religious coping strategies. The result of this process can be a transformation or conservation of the spiritual or religious orienting system.[29] It seems that mostly the content of religion and spirituality, that is, its implications on the belief system, can have a positive or negative effect on depression, not religion or spirituality itself. Therefore, there is only a limited scientific validity to measure the correlation between religion and depression, if there is no specification about the content of religious beliefs. Nevertheless, some specific patterns in the coping process are known to be associated with depression which are described below. Thus, religion and coping interact in a complex way: "some religious coping studies have reported nonsignificant, contradictory, or complex findings. [...] It is also possible that some forms of religious coping have mixed rather than exclusively positive or negative implications."[30] Scholars mostly assume that religion serves as a moderating variable between health and stress, and thus has direct and indirect effects on depression.[31]

27 Cf. also Huber's concept of centrality of religion, Stefan Huber and Odilo W. Huber, "The Centrality of Religiosity Scale (CRS)," *Religions* 3 (2012): 710–724.

28 Cf. Kenneth I. Pargament, Melissa D. Falb, Gene G. Ano and Amy B. Wachholtz, "The Religious Dimensions of Coping: Advances in Theory, Research, and Practice," in *Handbook of the Psychology of Religion and Spirituality*, eds. Raymond F. Paloutzian and Crystal L. Park (Princeton/New York: Guilford Press, 2013): 560–579.

29 Cf. Kenneth I. Pargament, *Spiritually integrated psychotherapy: Understanding and addressing the sacred* (New York: Guilford Press, 2007).

30 Pargament et al., "The Religious Dimensions of Coping," 560–579, 566.

31 Cf. Smith et al., "Religiousness and depression," 614–636.

3.2 Religious or Spiritual Struggles

Lately, religious and spiritual struggles have been in the focus of research on health and spirituality. Initiated by Pargament's results, researchers like Julie Exline point out the ambivalence of religious struggles that can either obscure religiosity but, on the other hand, may also transform someone's belief system into posttraumatic growth.[32] Whereas the research on religious coping has revealed a double-edged relationship between religion and mental health, it also becomes obvious that it may be difficult to clearly label religious coping in terms of 'positive' and 'negative'. Spiritual struggle focuses on "a form of distress or conflict in the religious or spiritual realm."[33] Such experiences have also been named as 'spiritual dryness',[34] 'religious conflicts', 'dark religious experiences'[35] and 'dark night'.[36] Different types of spiritual/religious struggles can be distinguished according to current studies: *transcendent forms* (related to the divine as a conflict or insecurity towards God; related to evil, demons or the devil as the experience to be tempted by the devil), *intrapersonal forms* (related to morality as e.g. unmoral action followed by guilt; related to the ultimate meaning in life, e.g. doubting the worth and importance of one's life; related to doubt as questioning religious beliefs) and finally *struggles in interpersonal relationships* (such as conflicts with people, groups or institutions related to religion or spirituality).[37] In the study of Exline et al., depression was more related to divine

---

32 Cf. Julie J. Exline and Erich D. Rose, "Religious and Spiritual Struggles," in *Handbook of the Psychology of Religion and Spirituality*, eds. Raymond F. Paloutzian and Crystal L. Park (New York: Guilford Press, 2013): 380–398. German version: Julie J. Exline and Erich D. Rose, "Religiöse und spirituelle Konflikte," in *Religiosität: Die dunkle Seite: Beiträge zur empirischen Religionsforschung*, eds. Christian Zwingmann, Constantin Klein and Florian Jeserich (Münster/New York: Waxmann, 2017): 65–90.

33 Julie J. Exline, "Religious and Spiritual Struggles," in *APA Handbook of Psychology, Religion, and Spirituality. Vol. 1: Context, Theory, and Research*, ed. Kenneth Pargament (Washington D.C.: American Psychological Association, 2013): 459–475, 460.

34 Arndt Büssing, Jochen Sautermeister, Eckard Frick and Klaus Baumann, "Reactions and Strategies of German Catholic Priests to Cope with Phases of Spiritual Dryness," *Journal of Religion and Health* 56(3) (2017): 1018–1031.

35 Christian Zwingmann, Constantin Klein and Florian Jeserich (eds.), *Religiosität: Die dunkle Seite: Beiträge zur empirischen Religionsforschung* (Münster/New York: Waxmann, 2017).

36 Regina Bäumer and Michael Plattig (eds.), *‚Dunkle Nacht' und Depression* (Ostfildern: Grünewald, 2008).

37 Cf. Exline and Rose, "Religious and Spiritual Struggles," 380–398.

38 Cf. Julie J. Exline, Kenneth I. Pargament., Joshua B. Grubbs and Anne Marie Yali, "The Religious and Spiritual Struggles Scale: Development and initial validation," *Psychology of Religion and Spirituality* 6(3) (2014): 208–222.

struggle and struggling with ultimate meaning. Doubt on the other hand, predicted more distress but was associated with less depression afterwards.[38] Thus, religious struggles and depression seem to be intertwined: on the one hand, religious struggles can predict depression, but depression also can come along with spiritual/religious struggle. In a prospective study, non-strugglers, chronic strugglers and transitory strugglers were identified, and the study came to the conclusion that only chronic versions are supposedly disadvantageous for mental health.[39] Another study points out that experiencing more stressful events may increase spiritual/religious struggle, if there are more negative emotions (e.g. anger or death anxiety) and social isolation, or an insecure relationship with God.[40] Lately, research about spiritual/religious struggles has also gained attention in a European and German context.[41] In a recent Swiss study by Fitchett et al., similar findings have been replicated, indicating that divine struggles correlate with more depression and anxiety, and were reported to at least some extent in nearly half of the sample of medically hospitalized patients. Patients that felt punished or abandoned by God during their illness, had higher levels of anxiety and depression.[42]

3.3 Other Variables Mediating the Relationship between Depression and Religion or Spirituality

Some other variables are influencing the relationship between mental health and religion and spirituality. Personality characteristics like neuroticism, optimism, need of control or self-esteem seem to highly interact with depression

---

39 Cf. Kenneth I. Pargament, Harold G. Koenig, Nalini Tarakeshwar and June Hahn, "Religious Coping Methods as Predictors of Psychological, Physical and Spiritual Outcomes among Medically Ill Elderly Patients: A Two-year Longitudinal Study," *Journal of Health Psychology* 9(6) (2004): 713–730.

40 Cf. Kelly M. Trevino, Kenneth I. Pargament, Neal Krause, Gail Ironson, and Peter Hill, "Stressful Events and Religious/Spiritual Struggle: Moderating Effects of the General Orienting System," *Psychology of Religion and Spirituality* (2017): https://doi.org/10.1037/rel0000149 (last accessed on 1 April 2020).

41 E.g. cf. Christian Zwingmann, Constantin Klein and Florian Jeserich, *Religiosität: Die dunkle Seite. Beiträge zur empirischen Religionsforschung* (Münster/New York: Waxmann, 2017). See also the project at the University of Bern: https://www.religious-conflicts.unibe.ch (last accessed on 1 April 2020; Isabelle Noth and Jessica Lampe, "Spiritual Struggles," in Encyclopedia of Psychology and Religion, ed. David A. Leeming (Berlin/Heidelberg: Springer, 2019), 1–4.

42 Cf. George Fitchett, Urs Winter-Pfändler and Kenneth I. Pargament, "Struggle with the divine in Swiss patients visited by chaplains: prevalence and correlates," *Journal of Health Psychology* 19(8) (2014): 966–976.

and religion and thus moderate the relationship. Neuroticism seems to predict the strongest interaction with depression – which is no surprise, since one of the subscales of neuroticism measures depressive symptoms – and religious involvement is related to less neuroticism, more often showing no significant relationship.[43] Also, gender is often shown to have an impact on the relationship between depression and religion. Women are more often engaged in religious activities, and also are more affected by depressive moods.[44] Another important variable is age. Braam showed that older people are not only more religious but also their faith is more affected during a depressive episode – this might be due to the higher salience of religion in their orienting system. Additionally, physical problems, which occur more often during higher age, also influence the relationship.[45] Other variables can be norms and values which are rooted in the orienting system together with religious convictions of the specific denomination and community. Finally, the severity of depression is relevant, too. Whereas religion may help during mild phases of depressive moods with only a few symptoms, during heavy episodes, it may be impossible or very difficult to continue practicing religion or keep up faith.[46]

4 Religious and Depressive Phenomena

As has been made clear already, religion and depression form a complex relationship. In the following, some characteristic phenomena will be described. As they are always intertwined, we will speak of associations and correlations instead of causalities.

43 Cf. Koenig et al., *Handbook of religion and health*, 145–173, 166.

44 There are different coping styles regarding depression. Tendentiously, more males cope through activities and substance abuse, women through emotional regulation and religion, cf. J. Angst, A. Gamma, M. Gastpar, J.-P. Lépine, J. Mendlewicz and A. Tylee, "Gender differences in depression. Epidemiological findings from the European DEPRES I and II studies," *European archives of psychiatry and clinical neuroscience* 252(5) (2002): 201–209. There are gender differences for prayer and church attendance (cf. details below), Joanna Maselko, R. David Hayward, Alexandra Hanlon, Stephen Buka and Keith Meador, "Religious service attendance and major depression: A case of reverse causality?," *American journal of epidemiology* 175(6) (2012): 576–583; For gender and race cf. R. T. Petts and Anne Joliff, "Religion and Adolescent Depression: The Impact of Race and Gender," *Review of Religious Research* 49(4) (2008): 395–414.

45 Cf. Aarjan W. Braam, Martin J. Prince and Aartjan T. Beekman et al., "Physical health and depressive symptoms in older Europeans. Results from EURODEP," *The British journal of psychiatry* 187 (2005): 35–42.

46 Cf. explanations for different phenomena below.

4.1 Image of God and Self-Esteem

A crucial factor, at least in monotheistic religions, has been the focus on the image of God in depression research. Alienation and distance from God is a burden that comes with depression. The image of God and self-esteem are highly interrelated. Seeing God as loving, supporting, and friendly correlates with a higher self-esteem, the opposite is true for perceiving God as cruel and punishing.[47] Because self-worth usually is low during a depressive episode, the image of God can be affected as well, resulting in doubt, spiritual struggles, or a darkened, absent God. On the other hand, thinking about God as distant or punishing can be associated with other symptoms of depression.[48]

In a German context, the concept of 'ecclesial induced neurosis' ('ekklesiogene Neurose') was popular during the 1980s and 1990s and assumed that images of a powerful, controlling and punishing God were implemented according to church dogmas.[49] Current perspectives propose to dismiss this approach because the image of God is multifactorial and there is no monocausal relation between the two factors.[50] Braam et al. found for a sample of older patients in a longitudinal survey that chronical depression is associated with an image of God of fear, the feeling of being wronged by God, or negative religious coping.[51] This points to the crucial role of feelings towards God concerning depression and the factor of age. Because many older patients may have experienced negative images of God

---

47 Cf. Leslie J. Francis, Harry M. Gibson and Mandy Robbins, "God images and self-worth among adolescents in Scotland," *Mental Health, Religion & Culture* 4(2) (2001): 103–108.

48 For a summary on the negative image of God cf. Anton A. Bucher, "Zornig und strafend – oder zu milde? Negative Gottesbilder," in *Religiosität: Die dunkle Seite: Beiträge zur empirischen Religionsforschung*, eds. Christian Zwingmann, Constantin Klein and Florian Jeserich (Münster/New York: Waxmann, 2017): 23–42.

49 Very influential in Germany was Tilman Moser's book about the God intoxication, *Gottesvergiftung* (Frankfurt am Main: Suhrkamp, 1976).

50 Cf. Christian Zwingmann, Constantin Klein and Florian Jeserich,"Ekklesiogene Neurose," in *Religiosität: Die dunkle Seite: Beiträge zur empirischen Religionsforschung*, eds. Christian Zwingmann, Constantin Klein and Florian Jeserich (Münster/New York: Waxmann, 2017): 43–64.

51 Cf. Aarjan W. Braam, Hanneke Schaap-Jonker and Marleen H. L. van der Horst et al., "Twelve-year history of late-life depression and subsequent feelings to God," *The American journal of geriatric psychiatry* 22(11) (2014): 1272–1281. They used the translated questionnaire developed by Murken and colleagues, Sebastian Murken, Katja Möschl, Claudia Müller and Claudia Appel, "Entwicklung und Validierung der Skalen zur Gottesbeziehung und zum religiösen Coping," in *Spiritualität transdisziplinär: Wissenschaftliche Grundlagen im Zusammenhang mit Gesundheit und Krankheit*, eds. Arndt Büssing and Niko Kohls (Berlin: Springer, 2011): 75–90.

in their religious education, they are more likely to suffer from religiously induced emotions like fear, anxiety, and depressed mood.[52] People that are feeling punished by God show higher levels of depression.[53] An important observation is that the image of God and its influence on mental health is highly correlated with the amount of perceived control and action in life.

Depression also comes along with a negative focus on the self. If the individual's self-image is full of negative aspects, this may lead to a feeling of worthlessness, feeling small and insignificant, and consequently this impression could be reinforced by an image of God that puts power and control alone in the hands of God. Whereas some individuals may feel powerless and small and accordingly are passive and helpless, this is associated with more depressive symptoms.[54] On the contrary, people with collaborative coping styles, who interact with God as a partner and cope actively at the same time, experience less depression.[55] In their study, Greenway and colleagues examined that self-liking strongly predicted God being seen positively. Especially women with a positive self-concept, saw God more positively and had lower rates of depression. If they felt God's presence in their lives, they also had a better relationship to themselves. People with higher depression rates perceived God as caring less for them and also had less self-esteem and feeling of self-competence. Thus, personality characteristics and self-perception may be influenced by the image of God (and vice versa), resulting in outcomes for mental health.[56] Interestingly, an ambivalent image of God that contains multi-fold characteristics is more helpful in times of stress than a narrow image of an only loving and caring God that does not include ways to address problems and pain – and this can be as problematic as focusing on negative aspects.[57] However, if the perception of God turns out to

---

52 Cf. Bucher, "Zornig und strafend – oder zu milde?" 23–42, 26–27.

53 Cf. Stacy C. Parenteau, Nancy A. Hamilton, Wei Wu, Kevin Latinis, Lori B. Waxenberg and Mary Y. Brinkmeyer, "The mediating role of secular coping strategies in the relationship between religious appraisals and adjustment to chronic pain: The middle road to Damascus," *Social Indicators Research* 104 (2011): 407–425.

54 God-mediated control and self-responsibility thus interact and are also associated with culture. Cf. Richard D. Hayward and Neal Krause, "Trajectories of late-life change in God-mediated control," *The journals of gerontology. Series B, Psychological sciences and social sciences* 68(1) (2013): 49–58.

55 Cf. Kenneth I. Pargament, "Religion and the Problem-Solving Process: Three Styles of Coping," *Journal for the Scientific Study of Religion* 27(1) (1988): 90–104.

56 Cf. Philip A. Greenway, Lisa C. Milne and Veronica Clarke, "Personality variables, self-esteem and depression and an individual's perception of God," *Mental Health, Religion & Culture* 6(1) (2003): 45–58.

57 Cf. Pargament, *Spiritually integrated psychotherapy*, 138.

be too ambiguous and contradicting, this can also result in internal conflicts like an ambivalent relationship to the sacred, self-degradation, or demonization of the self and others.[58] Since the image of God may be reflecting on the self, Klessmann also argues, that negative images of God are a mirror of biblical traditions, cultural background and their individual adaption transported by education and biography, but in any case, they are only obscure shapes of the reality of the Holy. The image of God according to its rich tradition in the Bible and religious transmission, is ambivalent and has positive and negative aspects: love and passion, struggle and joy, suffering and healing. These have always been part of the religious experience of humankind and are thus to be taken into account when dealing with depression, too.[59]

4.2 Guilt and Shame

An additional criterion of depression can be the feeling of guilt, which can range from a mild form of being responsible for bad things by blaming oneself for minor incidents, up to a delusion of guilt which only happens in a minority of depressive individuals.[60] Roughly spoken, there are two types of guilt: appropriate and maladaptive guilt.[61] In most cases, maladaptive guilt and shame result from depression and thus are symptoms of the illness. In empirical studies, it was shown that greater levels of guilt and feeling alienated by God were associated with greater levels of depression and suicidality.[62] Guilt and shame can also result from the experience of being distant or disconnected from God or during spiritual struggles.[63] Depressed persons sometimes felt they had committed an unforgivable sin, and

58 Cf. Pargament, *Spiritually integrated psychotherapy*, 143–149.

59 Cf. Michael Klessmann, "Pastoralpsychologische Seelsorge mit depressiven Menschen," in *Pastoralpsychologische Perspektiven in der Seelsorge: Grenzgänge zwischen Theologie und Psychologie*, ed. Michael Klessmann (Göttingen: Vandenhoeck & Ruprecht, 2017): 27–42, 48 and 34.

60 Cf. Gabriele Stotz-Ingenlath and Eckard Frick, "Depressives Schulderleben: Symptomatologie und Diagnostik," *Schweizer Archiv für Neurologie und Psychiatrie* 157(3) (2006): 94–102.

61 Cf. June P. Tangney and Ronda L. Daering, *Shame and guilt* (New York: Guilford Press, 2004).

62 Cf. Elizabeth J. Albertsen, Lynn E. O'Connor and Jack W. Berry, "Religion and interpersonal guilt: Variations across ethnicity and spirituality," *Mental Health, Religion and Culture* 9(1) (2006): 67–84.

63 Cf. Kelly Murray and Joseph W. Ciarrocchi, "The dark side of Religion, Spirituality and the moral emotions: shame, guilt, and negative religiosity as markers for life dissatisfaction," *Journal of Pastoral Counseling* 42 (2007): 22–41.

then interpret their feelings of guilt religiously.[64] Maladaptive guilt can also occur during a physical illness like cancer, if religious individuals are attributing the cause of their illness to their misdemeanours, and therefore develop depressive symptoms.[65] Thus, religious guilt or the impression of having sinned against God can point to depression and is merely a symptom of the illness itself. Religious mind-sets and values can create high internal norms and standards which can be understood as religious schemata. These can create conflicts between the will to practice religion and the will to believe, but not being able to follow and fulfil all standards the way someone feels he or she is supposed to.[66] This conflict leads to the feeling of guilt. To offer confession and absolution from a religious perspective is, therefore, not helfpful. On the contrary, it can increase the feeling of guilt by convincing the depressed person that his or her feeling of guilt is justified and real.[67]

4.3 Religion, Suicidality, and Depression

Suicidality is an additional criterion for depression being a highly complex phenomenon that also occurs across different psychiatric diagnoses. It, however, can also exist without depression or any psychiatric abnormalities. Also, suicidality is best described as a continuum from tendencies to real action.[68] In monotheistic religions like Judaism, Christianity or Islam, suicide is prohibited

---

64 Cf. Julie J. Exline, Ann Marie Yali and William C. Sanderson, "Guilt, Discord and Alienation: The Role of Religious Strain in Depression and Suicidality," *Journal of Clinical Psychology* 56(2) (2000): 1481–1496. The unforgiveable sin is considered the sin against the Holy Spirit that will not be forgiven. In some religious, mostly evangelical contexts, the fear of that kind of sin is common. Cf. Anton Bucher, *Die dunkle Seite der Kirche* (Etsdorf: Galia, 2010).

65 This has been shown in an Iranian study with Muslims, Seyedeh Z. Alavi, Forogh Amin and Azar P. Savoji, "Relationship between Pathological Guilt and God Image with Depression in Cancer Patients," *Procedia – Social and Behavioral Sciences* 84 (2013): 919–924.

66 Cf. Koenig et al., *Handbook of religion and health*, 148.

67 Cf. Jörg Bade, *Depression und Segen. Zur seelsorgerlichen Begegnung mit depressiven Menschen* (Münster: Lit Verlag, 2000), 329–330. Bade instead suggests to offer a blessing instead of the repenting ceremony because it symbolizes the unquestioning nature of God's blessing.

68 Cf. Annette Haußmann, "Suizidalität und Depression," in *Menschen mit Depression. Orientierungen und Impulse für die Praxis in Kirchengemeinden*, eds. Birgit Weyel and Beate Jakob (Gütersloh: Gütersloher Verlagshaus, 2014): 36–44; Bart van den Brink, Hanneke Schaap and Aarjan W. Braam, "Moral Objections and Fear of Hell: An Important Barrier to Suicidality," *Journal of Religion and Health* 57 (2018): 2301–2312.

because it is considered a sin and therefore forbidden or highly stigmatized.[69] Several studies have shown that the higher the religiosity and the more important religion is in a certain country, the lower the suicidal rates.[70] This robust finding is presented in various reviews and it seems clear that religiosity functions as a barrier to suicide, regardless of denomination.[71] Dervic et al. examined the relationship between religiosity, depression and suicidal behavior. They found that although nonreligious and religious participants were hopeless and depressed to the same degree and shared the same burden concerning life event induced distress, people with religious belief had fewer suicidal ideas and suicide attempts.[72] Later, they found that in bipolar patients, only the number of suicidal attempts was related to religious moral objections, but there was no relationship to suicidal ideas.[73]

The mechanism seems to be that religion not only offers a way to see the future with hope but also offers a new perspective and meaning in life.[74] The belief in afterlife is relevant to most religious traditions and also some spiritual attitudes. One crucial criterion for diagnosing a depressive episode, is hopelessness and the darkening of the future. But moral restrictions on suicide are probably more powerful barriers blocking suicidal tendencies in a manner which hinders suicidal ideas from shifting to suicidal actions. Van den Brink and Braam showed that moral objections to suicide may prevent suicidal action, as fear of hell is a powerful belief that impedes suicide.[75] Most of the highly religious people believe in life after death and some also in hell, especially Catholics or orthodox Protestants, but there are also significant differences

---

69 Buddhism and Hinduism are also against suicide, but have a softer mind-set towards suicide, and some traditions in Hinduism, explicitly allow suicide, particularly that of a woman who follows her husband into death. Cf. Erminia Colucci and Graham Martin, "Religion and spirituality along the suicidal path," *Suicide Life Threat Behavior* 38 (2008): 229–244.

70 Cf. Raphael M. Bonelli, "Suizid und Religiosität," in *Psychotherapie und Spiritualität: Mit existenziellen Konflikten und Transzendenzfragen professionell umgehen*, eds. Michael Utsch, Raphael M. Bonelli and Samuel Pfeifer (Berlin/Heidelberg: Springer, 2014): 133–142, 135–136.

71 Cf. Koenig et al., *Handbook of religion and health*, 174–190, and Harold Koenig and Raphael Bonelli, "Mental disorders, religion and spirituality 1990 to 2010: a systematic evidence based review," *Journal of Religion and Health 52* (2013): 657–673.

72 Cf. Dervic et al., "Religious affiliation and suicide attempt," *American Journal of Psychiatry* 161 (2004): 2303–2308.

73 Cf. Dervic et al., "Moral or religious objections to suicide may protect against suicidal behavior in bipolar disorder," *The Journal of Clinical Psychiatry* 72(10) (2011): 1390–1396.

74 Cf. Steven Stack, "Religiosity, depression, and suicide," in *Religion and mental health*, ed. John F. Schumaker (Oxford/New York: Oxford University Press, 1992): 87–98.

75 Cf. van den Brink et al, "Moral Objections and Fear of Hell," 2301–2312.

among denomination to be considered.[76] This again points to the importance of distinguishing the contents of religious beliefs. But it also raises another question: Religion, in this case, does not eliminate suicidal thoughts. Instead, it raises fear and thus may increase burden and despair even further. Once more, the ambivalent constellation between the two variables becomes obvious: religiosity may help to save someone's life, but it takes more to recover from suicidal thoughts than just developing a different perspective on life. Whether religion can offer a resource to reduce such thoughts, depends largely on the individual's image of God, their norms and values, their personal religious orienting system – and an appropriate psychotherapeutic treatment of depression as well.

4.4 Social Problems in the Realm of the Religious Community

According to Aaron Beck, depression is accompanied by three main cognitive distortions: the self, the future and the world so that other people can only be seen in a negative light.[77] Fellow human beings, even those who normally support the individual and share his or her beliefs, are seen as distant or hostile during a depressive episode. Therefore, social problems may arise also in a religious community. Distrust, misunderstandings, quarrels about religion and religious norms can appear in personal relationships and church congregations. It is therefore important to notice that this is a result of depression as an illness, not the bad will or aim of the depressive individual. Isolation within the religious community can result from depression, too.[78] This occurs due to at least three reasons. Firstly, people in the community may reject depressive persons simply because of their negative mood which is not easy to deal with. Secondly, there might be religious or spiritual reasons for isolating this person because he or she seems to threaten the belief system of the community by asking questions

---

76 Cf. Julie J. Exline, "Belief in heaven and hell among Christians in the United States: Denominational differences and clinical implications," *Journal of Death and Dying* 47(2) (2003): 155–168. There are also significant differences between denominational groups and their thoughts about afterlife. A qualitative study in Poland showed some significant differences in beliefs between Protestants and Catholics concerning hell and heaven. Whereas Protestants mostly believed in hell as a place of being abandoned by God, Catholics talked more about hell as punishment and helplessness. Cf. Emilia Wroclawska-Warchala and Michal Warchala, "The heavens and hells we believe in. Individual eschatological Images as conditioned by denominational culture," *Archive for the psychology of religion* 37 (2015): 240–266.

77 Cf. Aaron T. Beck, *Cognitive therapy of depression* (Chichester: Wiley, 1979).

78 Cf. Annette Haußmann, "Einsamkeit und Spiritualität," in *Das Einsamkeitsbuch für Pflegeberufe*, ed. Thomas Hax-Schoppenhorst (Bern: Hogrefe, 2018): 153–163.

or articulating doubt about values, God or his presence.[79] Thirdly, the religious community could reject the depressed person because they are convinced that depression is a consequence of weak faith and or a veritable sign of God's punishment.[80] Although people can experience social support in their church community, conflict in the church network is associated with more depressive symptoms amongst their members.[81] Especially in religiously orthodox groups with high religious norms and rigid belief systems, depression rates were observed to be higher than in the normal population.[82] There are also hints that such groups may conceal their depressive symptoms because religious struggling is considered normal and depression therefore is misunderstood as a religious challenge.[83] Either way, isolation from the religious community further lowers social support, which is much needed in times of crisis.

5 Preventive and Buffering Functions of Religion

As studies have indicated, religion can play a buffering role as a resource during depression and furthermore can also prevent depressive episodes.[84] It is also necessary to highlight the ambivalent relationship once more: relying on religion as a resource does not mean that this resource is always available

---

79 Cf. Koenig et al., *Handbook of religion and health*, 148.

80 Cf. Braam et al., "Religious climate and geographical distribution of depressive symptoms in older Dutch citizens," *Journal of Affective Disorders* 54(1–2) (1999): 149–159.

81 Cf. Linda M. Chatters, Robert J. Taylor, Amanda T. Woodward and Emily J. Nicklett, "Social support from church and family members and depressive symptoms among older African Americans," *The American journal of geriatric psychiatry* 23(6) (2015): 559–567.

82 Higher depression rates were found in members of pietist groups in the Netherlands, cf. Braam et al., "Religious climate and geographical distribution," 149–159. A higher depression rate was measured in members of Jehovas Witnesses in Maria C. Norton, Archana Singh and Ingmar Skoog, "Church attendance and new episodes of major depression in a community study of older adults: The Cache County Study," *The journals of gerontology / B* 63(3) (2008): 129–137.

83 Cf. A. A. de Lely, Walter W. van den Broek, Paul G. Mulder and Tom K. Birkenhäger, "Symptomen bij een depressie; bevindelijk gereformeerde versus niet-kerkelijke patiënten [Symptoms of depression in strict Calvinist patients and in patients without religious affiliations: a comparison]," *Tijdschrift voor psychiatrie* 51(5) (2009): 279–289.

84 Cf. Braam, "Religion und Depression," 273–290, 275. Also for a more general model of mental health and religion cf. Constantin Klein and Cornelia Albani, "Religiosität und psychische Gesundheit – empirische Befunde und Erklärungsansätze," in *Gesundheit – Religion – Spiritualität, Befunde und Erklärungsansätze*, eds. Constantin Klein, Hendrik Berth and Friedrich Balck (Weinheim: Juventa, 2011): 215–245.

during different phases in life. It also can be hidden or inaccessible during times of stress. What determines 'good' coping therefore depends on the individual, their resources, the context and particular situation, and the severity of the depressive symptoms.[85] But it should be mentioned that some resources *can* help to reduce and prevent depression, and therefore support the observation that religious people who depend on the content of their religiosity can cope better. Overall, three predisposing factors support a better recovery from depression, thus buffering depressive symptoms: intrinsic religious motivation, the salience of religion for the individual, and positive religious coping.[86] Also religious practice and participation in congregational life may help a depressed person as discussed in the following.

5.1 Prayer and Meditation

Prayer is a frequently chosen way to cope with negative feelings. The first positive influence of prayer is that sorrow and problems can be articulated. This also means that the individual can express him or herself and what bothers him or her. A lot of mental problems arise because the problem is not realized and emotions cannot be felt or dealt with. Thus, praying is one way to cope with problems. People pray more often than they participate in other religious rituals like Sunday services. Even people who are not part of a religious community or not explicitly religious are praying. During distressing times people pray more often and they often use this strategy successfully to cope with pain and suffer less from depressive symptoms.[87] During a depressive episode, even some nonreligious people may turn to God, although some studies reported more depressive symptoms in nonreligious patients that pray, especially in those who are widowed.[88] This may indicate that prayer serves as a coping strategy also for those who are not religious, if they suffer from a high level of distress.[89]

---

85 Cf. Pargament, *The Psychology of Religion and Coping.*

86 Cf. Braam, "Religion und Depression," 273–290, 281.

87 Cf. Gerhard Andersson, "Chronic pain and praying to a higher power. Useful or useless?", *Journal of Religion and Health* 47 (2008): 176–187.

88 Cf. Aarjan W. Braam, Dorly J. Deeg, Jan L. Poppelaars, Aartjan T. Beekman and Willem van Tilburg, "Prayer and depressive symptoms in a period of secularization: Patterns among older adults in the Netherlands," *The American journal of geriatric psychiatry* 15(4) (2007): 273–281.

89 Cf. the interpretation of Braams study in Koenig et al., *Handbook of religion and health,* 145–173, 160.

During a depressive episode, lack of concentration and doubts regarding the relationship with God make praying difficult. A lot of depressed people describe that they not only feel distant to God, but also feel that he is not answering prayers, or that they are simply not able to pray anymore.[90] It is very helpful for ill people to know that these difficulties are rather a result of their illness and have nothing to do with personal failure or being abandoned by God. Also, the burden can be reduced by telling them that God is still there, although the individual does not feel this presence. Furthermore, praying is not explicitly a duty of the religious individual and it is not a sin to not pray if one is not able to do so. This might be the reason why some studies do not show significant associations between the frequency of praying and depression.[91] Interestingly, in some studies, different types of prayer have shown influence on depressive symptoms. Whereas small negative effects on depression were found for adoration prayer and receptive prayer, moderate negative effects were observed for praying for the well-being of others, but that was also partially influenced by social support. Prayers of thanksgiving were most difficult for depressed individuals. Although there was less depression associated with prayers of thanksgiving, this effect was fully moderated by meditation.[92] This again indicates the difficulty of religious activities during depression that sometimes hinders people in prayer. Also, there is an interesting distinction concerning feelings and actions towards God. Whereas only anger towards God predicts higher levels of distress, elements of prayer like complaining, arguing or questioning lead to less depression or distress.[93] In the longitudinal study of Hayward et al., prayer was found to mediate the relationship between subjective religiousness and a better outcome with less post-treatment depression. Thus, individuals who pray more often are not necessarily less depressive, but show a better recovery after therapy.[94]

90 Cf. Pfeifer, "Seelenfinsternis und dunkle Nacht der Seele," 121–132, and cf. chapter II.3 in this volume: Beate Jakob, *Is Faith a Source of Strength? Do Congregations offer Support? A Qualitative Study with People Affected by Mental Disorders and Their Relatives*.

91 Cf. Braam et al, "Prayer and depressive symptoms in a period of secularization," 273–281.

92 Cf. John E. Pérez, Amy R. Smith, Rebecca L. Norris, Katia M. Canenguez, Elizabeth F. Tracey and Susan B. DeCristofaro, "Types of prayer and depressive symptoms among cancer patients: The mediating role of rumination and social support," *Journal of behavioral medicine* 34(6) (2011): 519–530.

93 Cf. Julie J. Exline, Steven J. Krause and Karen A. Broer, "Spiritual Struggle Among Patients Seeking Treatment for Chronic Headaches: Anger and Protest Behaviors Toward God," *Journal of Religion and Health* 55(5) (2016): 1729–1747.

94 Cf. David R. Hayward, Amy D. Owen, Harold G. Koenig, David C. Steffens and Martha E. Payne, "Longitudinal relationships of religion with posttreatment depression severity in older

Studies have, however, also indicated that praying during a severe depressive episode does not show a significant positive effect on depression, or can even increase the depressive symptoms.[95] Praying during times of struggle is an existential experience[96] and it can also be useful to stop religious practice for a time in severe episodes instead of increasing hopelessness. Even in the Bible, there are ancient prayers talking about a distant God, especially in the Book of Lamentations. The reality of suffering is part of the trustworthy relationship between God and the praying human and it reflects on the dynamic relationship between God and creation as it is expressed in the Psalms – from lamentation and complaining to worship. Praying – from a theological perspective – thus is a dynamic interaction that goes beyond emotional regulation by expressing feelings and doubts. However, it expresses the reliance on God's help and trust in Him, although he might be perceived as distant in times of depression and prayer may then also temporarily lose its purpose and solace.[97]

Meditation is a spiritual practice, which not necessarily includes belief in God, but nevertheless can help to reduce depressive symptoms.[98] Predominantly, a Buddhism inspired approach of mindfulness is currently used in depression therapy and considered useful also for atheists or in secular contexts.[99] The central concept is the focus on the inner self and a shifted attention to one's feelings and thoughts without judging them immediately. Different types of yoga and meditation have proven to be effective against depressive symptoms and dysthymia.[100]

psychiatric patients: Evidence of direct and indirect effects," *Depression research and treatment* (2012): 1–8.

95 Cf. Braam et al, "Prayer and depressive symptoms in a period of secularization," 273–281.

96 Cf. from a biblical perspective Ralph Kunz, "Beten in der Anfechtung," in *Gebet als Resonanzereignis. Annäherungen im Horizont von Spiritual Care,* ed. Simon Peng-Keller (Göttingen: Vandenhoeck & Ruprecht, 2017): 159–192.

97 Cf. Arndt Büssing, "Empirische Zugänge zum Beten," in *Gebet als Resonanzereignis. Annäherungen im Horizont von Spiritual Care,* ed. Simon Peng-Keller (Göttingen: Vandenhoeck & Ruprecht, 2017): 111–128, 126–127.

98 Cf. Amy B. Wachholtz and Elizabeth T. Austin, "Contemporary Spiritual Meditation: Practices and Outcomes," in *APA Handbook of Psychology, Religion, and Spirituality: Vol. 1: Context, Theory, and Research*, ed. Kenneth I. Pargament (Washington D.C: American Psychological Association, 2013): 311–327.

99 Cf. Jon Kabat-Zinn, "Mindfulness-based interventions in context: Past, present, and future," *Clinical Psychology: Science and Practice* 10 (2003): 144–156.

100 Cf. Lisa D. Butler et al., "Meditation with yoga, group therapy with hypnosis, and psychoeducation for long-term depressed mood: A randomized pilot trial," *Journal of Clinical Psychology* 64 (2008): 806–820 and Elisa H. Kozasa et al., "Evaluation of Siddha Samadhi Yoga for anxiety and depression symptoms: A preliminary study," *Psychological Reports* 103 (2008): 271–274.

Because it can buffer stress, meditation is also helpful to prevent depression.[101] The difference to praying is the dyadic relationship: Whereas people can address their sorrows and problems to a higher being, that is God, in praying, meditation does not require an explicitly religious framework and can also be useful for non-religious persons. Praying, however, is ambivalent in its effects on depression. It always depends on the image of God, the content of religious cognitions and the resulting emotions that determine whether prayer is helpful or harmful.

5.2 Church Attendance and Rituals

Church attendance is a factor, which has been most examined in religiosity since the beginning of research in psychology of religion. Whereas early studies indicated that church-goers had a health benefit, we now know that this is only one aspect of individual religiosity, and the positive effect of church attendance depends on various variables. Some studies with a prospective design have shown that attendance of religious services can prevent depression,[102] and that people attending services more frequently have a lower risk of depression and any lifetime mental disease.[103] There seems to be an U-shaped relationship between depression and church attendance. The deeper the depression, the less helpful is going to church, and some of the depressed are not able to follow their usual Sunday routine anymore.[104] For a protecting effect, not only the membership in a congregation, but the regular contact to others in a religious community seems to determine the influence on health. Maselko et al. proposed an inverse causal

---

101 Cf. Shauna L. Shapiro, Doug Oman, Carl E. Thoresen, Thomas G. Plante and Tim Flinders, "Cultivating mindfulness: Effects on well-being," *Journal of Clinical Psychology* 64 (2008): 840–862.

102 Cf. Yakov A. Barton, Lisa Miller, Priya Wickramaratne, Marc J. Gameroff and Myrna M. Weissman, "Religious attendance and social adjustment as protective against depression: A 10-year prospective study," *Journal of Affective Disorders* 146(1) (2013): 53–57. Also for a European context cf. Aarjan W. Braam, E. Hein, Dorly J. H. Deeg, J. W. R. Twisk, Aartjan T. Beekman and Willem van Tilburg, "Religious Involvement and 6-Year Course of Depressive Symptoms in Older Dutch Citizens: Results from the Longitudinal Aging Study Amsterdam," *Journal of Aging and Health* 16(4) (2004): 467–489.

103 Cf. Linda M. Chatters, Kai M. Bullard, Robert J. Taylor and Amanda T. Woodward et al., "Religious participation and DSM-IV disorders among older African Americans: Findings from the National Survey of American Life," *The American journal of geriatric psychiatry* 16(12) (2008): 957–965.

104 Cf. Robert J. Taylor, Linda M. Chatters and Ann W. Nguyen, "Religious participation and DSM IV major depressive disorder among Black Caribbeans in the United States," *Journal of immigrant and minority health* 15(5) (2013): 903–909.

relationship between depression and church attendance. Their results show that women with an onset of depression under 18 years are more likely to stop attending services, which is not the case for men.[105] These findings suggest that people, especially women, may stop attending services after the onset of depression and thus cannot profit from social support in church or public religious activities because they are no longer able to participate. Once more, it is important to note that the sort of congregation, the shared belief system, the social cohesion and the rules the social environment shares, determine the relationship between depression and religion. Thus, for mild depressive episodes, church attendance, hence meeting others, getting different impulses and seeing and hearing something new can be supportive for depressed people. But this is only true, if the environment is supporting, i.e. a caring but not judging community, with helpful others.

Rituals as opposed to conversations can happen without words. A blessing rather than offering repentance as a way to interact with God and receive unconditional love in the midst of darkness and suffering is helpful to depressive people.[106] Also, this is a good possibility for those who suffer from cognitive impairment during severe depressive episodes.

5.3 Forgiveness

Studies have shown that forgiveness to the self and to others can be helpful – especially in times of crisis and depression. Religion and spirituality encourage people to be more forgiving and generous towards others.[107] Current research indicates that self-forgiveness and the feeling of being forgiven by God have a significant correlation and are associated with less depressive symptoms.[108] Other studies found in a sample with older people that forgiveness of any kind, by God, of themselves, of others, mediated the relation between depression, well-being and religion.[109] Forgiveness can help to reduce the severity of depression and

105 Cf. Maselko et al. "Religious service attendance and major depression," 576–583.

106 Cf. Bade, *Depression und Segen*, 321–332.

107 Cf. Jessica M. Schultz, Benjamin A. Tallman and Elizabeth M. Altmaier, "Pathways to posttraumatic growth: The contributions of forgiveness and importance of religion and spirituality," *Psychology of Religion and Spirituality* 2 (2010): 104–114.

108 Cf. Alice M. Martin, *Exploring Forgiveness: The Relationship Between Feeling Forgiven by God and Self-Forgiveness for an Interpersonal Offense* (Electronic Thesis, 2008).

109 Cf. Kathleen A. Lawler-Row, "Forgiveness as a mediator of the religiosity-health relationship," *Psychology of Religion and Spirituality* 2 (2010): 1–16.

suicidality.[110] But as with other variables, it depends on the centrality of religion if there is a positive relationship between forgiveness by God and a forgivingness toward others.[111] Therefore it is safe to assume that highly religious people who believe in God's forgiveness can forgive themselves easier. Depressed persons often are rigid and strict towards themselves, suffering from high perfectionism, while showing low tolerance for mistakes they have made, paired with low self-esteem and self-acceptance. The mechanism behind the connection may be that hopelessness can be reduced by self-forgiving through gaining a different perspective on the self and can therefore function as a protective factor.[112] Toussaint et al. have suggested that being able to forgive oneself and others may protect against depression in a longitudinal perspective.[113] Some interventions have already been developed to reduce depression-related guilt by encouraging self-forgiveness.[114]

But there is also the notion that this feeling and perception of forgiveness takes some time and cannot be easily learned. Particularly depressive persons often have the problem of adequate emotional perception and regulation. Emotions of anger and disappointment can be hidden behind sadness and must first be acknowledged before encouraging forgiveness.[115] Initially, lamentation and sorrow are overtaking most of the inner space during a manifest depression. In the healing process, people can further explore and develop a

---

110 Cf. Jameson K. Hirsch, Jon R. Webb and Elizabeth L. Jeglic, "Forgiveness, depression, and suicidal behavior among a diverse sample of college students," *Journal of Clinical Psychology* 67(9) (2011): 896–906.

111 Cf. Stefan Huber, Mike Allemand and Odilo W. Huber, "Forgiveness by God and Human Forgivingness: The Centrality of the Religiosity Makes the Difference," *Archive for the Psychology of Religion* 33(1) (2011): 115–134.

112 Cf. Loren L. Toussaint, David R. Williams, Mike A. Musick and Susan A. Everson-Rose, "Why forgiveness may protect against depression: Hopelessness as an explanatory mechanism," *Personality and Mental Health*, 2(2) (2008): 89–103.

113 Cf. Loren L. Toussaint, Justin C. Marschall and David R. Williams, "Prospective associations between religiousness/spirituality and depression and mediating effects of forgiveness in a nationally representative sample of United States adults," *Depression Research and Treatment* (2012): 1–10.

114 Cf. Mickie L. Fisher and Julie J. Exline, "Moving toward self-forgiveness: Removing barriers related to shame, guilt, and regret," *Social and Personality Psychology Compass* 4 (2010): 548–558.

115 Greenberg points out the importance to adequately deal with emotions in depression therapy and distinguishes secondary and primary emotions. Cf. Leslie S. Greenberg and Jeanne C. Watson, *Emotion-focused therapy for depression* (Washington DC: American Psychological Association, 2006).

sense of being forgiven and forgive themselves.[116] The connection to acceptance and tolerance of one's own self is close to forgiveness. Also, this variable is not static but dynamic in nature, resulting in change over time as a relational construct.[117] Again, this factor corresponds with the individual's image of God.[118] Furthermore, Exline and colleagues found that forgiveness is difficult if a person is angry towards God because God is considered responsible for bad experiences or is perceived as cruel or abandoning.[119] On the contrary, a more collaborative relationship with God seems to support forgiveness for others and oneself.[120] If the image of God is stable and resilient against anger, questions and doubts, religious struggles can also help the relationship to grow: "resilient relationships with God often include some tolerance for protest in form of anger, questioning, and complaint – just so long as exiting the relationship is not seen as a viable option."[121]

German studies have shown the power of forgiveness in several contexts and the salience of forgiveness especially for highly religious persons.[122] It must, however, be noted that forgiveness cannot be automatically used as a kind of coping tool, but rather, self-forgiveness through religious forgiving by God can offer a way of gaining new self-esteem and working on one's image of God in an ongoing process.

---

116 Cf. Robert D. Enright, *Vergebung als Chance: Neuen Mut fürs Leben finden* (Bern: Hogrefe, 2006). Enright points to the importance of first expressing anger towards the problem or person and afterwards encouraging forgiveness.

117 Cf. Everett Worthington Jr., Don E. Davis, Joshua N. Hook, Daryl R. van Tongeren, Aubrey L. Gartner, David J. Jennings II, Chelsea L. Greer and Yin Lin, "Religion, Spirituality, and Forgiveness," in *Handbook of the psychology of Religion and Spirituality*, ed. Raymond F. Paloutzian and Crystal L. Park (New York: Guilford Press, 2015): 476–497.

118 Cf. Exline et al., "Guilt, Discord and Alienation," 1481–1496.

119 Cf. Julie J. Exline, Crystal L. Park, Joshua M. Smyth and Michael P. Carey, "Anger toward God: Social-cognitive predictors, prevalence, and links with adjustment to bereavement and cancer," *Journal of Personality and Social Psychology* 100(1) (2011): 129–148.

120 Cf. Daniel Escher, "How does religion promote forgiveness? Linking beliefs, orientations, and practices," *Journal for the Scientific Study of Religion* 52(1) (2013): 100–119.

121 Exline and Rose, "Religious and Spiritual Struggles," 380–398, 387 and cf. also Julie J. Exline, Kalman J. Kaplan and Joshua B. Grubbs, "Anger exit and assertion: Do people see protest toward God as morally acceptable?," *Psychology of Religion and Spirituality* 4(4) (2012): 264–277.

122 Cf. Judith Lindner, "Einflüsse von Religiosität und Vergebung auf die psychische Gesundheit," *Wege zum Menschen* 68 (2016): 360–371.

5.4 Social Support

Participating in a religious or spiritual community, participating can be beneficial for mental health. Social support, therefore, is an important resource for mental health in various ways and especially for persons suffering from depression. Since isolation is a major danger, it helps to be a part of a social environment that offers group cohesion, comfort and material or emotional support. The congregation offers a social network that facilitates help-seeking behavior, a higher frequency of interacting with other people and receiving various types of social, emotional, spiritual or even material support.[123] Furthermore, the community also offers guidelines for living, a social identity that goes beyond social support itself because it is available even if the individual is not participating actively in the community.[124] But other studies have shown that regular participation increases social support over time which buffers negative health outcomes.[125] It also depends largely on the type of congregation, its cohesion and the type of support it can offer to the depressed person.[126] Particularly for those without family or close friends, a church congregation and their social support can be an important social network, which also notices differences in mood and behavior.[127] It may also be helpful if the congregation is informed about depression in general and how it can influence a person's religiosity and social behavior.[128] The knowledge that depression is a mental disorder that can

123 Different dimensions are supporting religious coping.

124 Cf. Crystal L. Park and Jeanne M. Slattery, "Religion, Spirituality, and Mental Health," in *Handbook of the Psychology of Religion and Spirituality*, eds. Raymond F. Paloutzian and Crystal L. Park (Princeton/New York: Guilford Press, 2013): 540–559, 548.

125 Cf. Cheryl L. Holt, David L. Roth, Jin Huang and Eddie M. Clark, "Role of religious social support in longitudinal relationships between religiosity and health-related outcomes in African Americans," *Journal of behavioral medicine* 41(1) (2018): 62–73.

126 For the differences between congregational culture and coping resources cf. Neal Krause and David R. Hayward, "Social Factors in the Church and Positive Religious Coping Responses: Assessing Differences Among Older Whites, Older Blacks, and Older Mexican Americans," *Review of Religious Research* 54(4) (2012): 519–541.

127 Cf. also the example of the choir leader that pointed out that the group noticed people missing or in depressed moods during rehearsals. Cf. chapter II.2 in this volume: Birgit Weyel, *What Motivates Volunteers in Congregations to Take Care of People with Mental Disorders? Looking at Pastoral Counselling Done by Volunteers in Local Congregations.*

128 Cf. Birgit Weyel and Beate Jakob, "Kirchengemeinden als soziales Netz und als Orte der Deutung von Gesundheit / Krankheit," in *Menschen mit Depression: Orientierungen und Impulse für die Praxis in Kirchengemeinden*, eds. Birgit Weyel and Beate Jakob (Gütersloh: Gütersloher Verlagshaus, 2014): 12–18.

affect anyone, brings tolerance and acceptance into the community and helps the affected person and their relatives and friends to open up and disclose themselves.

6 Spiritual Interventions in Psychotherapy and Pastoral Care

In addition to this short summary of resources, it has to be noted that other resources may be important as well. Among these are religious hope that goes beyond what is present at the very moment of suffering, a general sense of meaning in life, afterlife beliefs and various other individually shaped religious coping styles and strategies that can be discovered in qualitative research and in direct interaction.[129] Those resources cannot be discussed here, and there is need of further research. Therefore, I am now addressing the issue of how to embed spiritual resources in pastoral care and psychotherapy.

6.1 Approaches of Spiritual or Religious Therapy

Most of the approaches integrating spirituality or religion into (psycho)therapy have been developed in an US context. This is due to the role of religion in the US-American culture, but also because mental health professionals and religious leaders and ministers work together closely. In a European context, such approaches are labelled as 'Spiritual Care', 'existential interventions', or 'meaning-based therapy'. All these approaches perceive the individual as embedded in a broad framework of helpful resources to be relied on during mental illness, and they also understand health as a wide construct that includes the religious or spiritual dimension. It is worth mentioning some of these approaches. Kenneth Pargament offers a type of spiritually integrated therapy that deals with religious coping issues, especially with religious struggles. He addresses problems like 'small Gods' and 'false Gods', basically a form of work with the image of God and theodicy with the intention to broaden and deepen a client's relationship with the sacred. Also, internal religious or spiritual conflicts can

129 Cf. for a summary of more influencing factors Park and Slattery, "Religion, Spirituality, and Mental Health," 540–559. Some of those strategies we have identified in the qualitative study, presented chapter II.3 of this volume.

be part of the intervention.[130] John Peteet offers a framework to deal with depression and religiosity and therefore suggests three possibilities to address spiritual and religious issues. First, a therapist could limit his or her intervention strictly to the psychological dimension by focusing on a patients' internal or social problems. Secondly, spiritual and psychological aspects are both taken into account, including multi-professional work with pastors and psychotherapists or specific religiously or spiritually based programmes that deal with beliefs and emotions. Thirdly, the therapist can explicitly include the patient's religious or spiritual worldview and traditions and try to embed it into therapy.[131] Which of the approaches is appropriate depends on the needs of the patient and the therapist's knowledge and background.

Spiritually integrated therapy is called for particularly if patients are likely to develop some kind of pathological induced religiosity such as religious psychoses, or depressive religious guilt.[132] But it can also be useful to integrate spirituality and religion to some extent if this is important to the patient. Furthermore, questions of the meaning of life and existential questions may arise during therapy and thus therapists should also be able to deal with such issues. Also, in Germany there are some approaches that include spiritual and religious issues in depression therapy.[133] It is always important to be aware of the culture in which a certain religious or spiritual belief is embedded in.[134] In the US context, some

130 Cf. Pargament, *Spiritually integrated psychotherapy*, 276–292.

131 Cf. John R. Peteet, "Spiritually integrated treatment of depression: A conceptual framework," in *Depression research and treatment* (2012): 1–6. Cf. also John R. Peteet, *Depression and the soul: A guide to spiritually integrated treatment* (New York: Routledge, 2010).

132 Cf. the examples of Peter Kaiser, "Pathologische Religiosität im psychiatrischen Kontext," in *Religiosität: Die dunkle Seite: Beiträge zur empirischen Religionsforschung*, eds. Christian Zwingmann, Constantin Klein and Florian Jeserich (Münster/New York: Waxmann, 2017): 227–252 and cf. also Michael Utsch, *Pathologische Religiosität: Genese, Beispiele, Behandlungsansätze* (Stuttgart: Kohlhammer Verlag, 2012).

133 E.g. the depression programme of Reicherzer that is rooted in Marsha Linehans DBT-programme for borderline patients, cf. Markus Reicherzer, *Depressive Störungen: Differentielle manualisierte Behandlung mit Skillstraining und Psychoedukation* (Stuttgart: Schattauer GmbH Verlag für Medizin und Naturwissenschaften, 2017). For a more general approach of psychotherapy and spirituality cf. Eckhard Frick, Isgard Ohls, Gabriele Stotz-Ingenlath and Michael Utsch, eds., *Fallbuch Spiritualität in Psychotherapie und Psychiatrie* (Göttingen Vandenhoeck & Ruprecht, 2018).

134 Some background information about culture and spiritual care is given in Isabelle Noth, Emanuel Schweizer and Georg Wenz (eds.), *Pastoral and spiritual care across religions and cultures: Seelsorge und Spiritual Care in interkultureller Perspektive* (Göttingen/Bristol: Vandenhoeck & Ruprecht, 2017).

evaluation of spiritual care programmes within a psychotherapeutic context showed positive effects such as less harsh and punishing images of Gods and a more accepting relationship with God and the sacred, followed by less anxiety and depression.[135] Some possibilities to address spirituality and depression in therapy are given below[136]:

- *Assessing religion and spirituality*: A therapist should know if religious or spiritual beliefs and practices are important or relevant to the patient to some extent. Useful assessment or screening instruments can be used in clinical practice and in an outpatient context.[137]
- *Psychoeducation*: The therapist can explain the relationship between depression and religion, normalizing symptoms like guilt as a part of depression and religious guilt as resulting from depression, too; feeling lonely and not being able to pray can be the result of depression, and the image of God is affected and darkened due to depressive feelings like all other relationships. Also, it is important to clarify the relationship between depression and religion: Religious feelings are not responsible for the loss of faith, but loss of faith is a symptom of depression.
- *Challenging and changing religious schemata*: This type of mental intervention questions rigid and harsh beliefs about God and the world. Like other negative mind-sets, they can be restructured, although to some they might be perceived as sacred. Religious schemata are functioning as any other schema, producing automatic thoughts that can – if too negative – be changed into positive beliefs.
- *Working with emotions*: Negative and positive emotions regarding faith experiences, relationships to God or the sacred, people within the religious or spiritual community, and the view on the self, according to belief systems can be assessed and worked with.

---

135 Michael J. Thomas, Glendon L. Moriarty, Edward B. Davis and Elizabeth L. Anderson, "The Effects of a Manualized Group-Psychotherapy Intervention on Client God Images and Attachment to God: A Pilot Study," *Journal of Psychology and Theology* 39(1) (2011): 44–58.

136 I will only give some hints from cognitive behavioral therapy programmes that include spirituality and leave out the various psychodynamic approaches that are mentioned elsewhere.

137 Assessing spirituality or religion from a clinical perspective with cancer patients cf. Eckard Frick, Carola Riedner, Martin J. Fegg, S. Haufand and Gian D. Borasio, "A clinical interview assessing cancer patients' spiritual needs and preferences," *European Journal of Cancer Care* 15(3) (2006): 238–243; Carola Riedner and Thomas Hagen, "Spirituelle Anamnese," in *Spiritualität und Medizin. Gemeinsame Sorge für den kranken Menschen (Münchner Reihe Palliative Care 4)*, eds. Eckhard Frick and Traugott Roser (Stuttgart [2]2011): 234–241.

- *Talking about meaning in life*: Since meaning making is important to everyone, it is relevant in therapy, too. By carefully assessing someone's 'must haves' in life and constituents of meaning, religious or spiritual beliefs and practices can be addressed.[138]

6.2 Pastoral Care and Depression

It is important for pastoral care workers to notice a depressed person in the first place. Depression is an illness, not a sign for little or weak belief in God. Therefore, it is also important to mention that depression is treatable and can be cured the faster the person gets therapeutic help. On the other hand, some people believe that their mental disorder is due to God's punishment or a result for not enough believing in God or failing to following spiritual or religious rules. It could help to point out that due to depression, many people think that they have lost their hope and faith, but that hope and faith – as well as other aspects in life – will come back eventually after a successful treatment of depression. For some, a minister represents the sacred and God, and therefore expectations can be high – especially if the minister tries to fulfil them completely.[139] Depressive people sometimes cannot get help for themselves actively. They need someone to approach them and look at their needs, including spiritual needs, and point out possibilities for further treatment. Therefore, an outreaching pastoral care is a way to bring help to those who most need it, like home visits to older ones, caregiving relatives, patients in nursing homes or hospitals. Some persons need to be encouraged to talk about problems and need some time to start talking about difficulties and sorrows. This is because they are convinced they do not deserve help because they themselves are guilty for their situation, or because they think no one can help them.[140] In addition, it is important to also include relatives and family members in the multi-professional helping system

138 Cf. Tatjana Schnell, *Psychologie des Lebenssinns* (Berlin: Springer, 2016). For a critical perspective cf. Michael Utsch, „Ausschluss oder Einbeziehung spiritueller Interventionen?", in *Psychotherapie und Spiritualität: Mit existenziellen Konflikten und Transzendenzfragen professionell umgehen*, eds. Michael Utsch, Raphael M. Bonelli and Samuel Pfeifer (Berlin/Heidelberg: Springer, 2014): 111–120.

139 Cf. Klessmann, "Pastoralpsychologische Seelsorge mit depressiven Menschen," 27–42, 28.

140 Cf. Christoph Morgenthaler, *Seelsorge*, Lehrbuch Praktische Theologie, Vol. 3 (Gütersloh: Gütersloher Verlagshaus 2009), 187.

of pastoral care.[141] Knowledge about depression and about one's self and one's own mechanisms of coping and religion is crucial to a successful pastoral care.[142] Klaus Depping describes three possibilities to deal with depressed older people according to CBT-related, humanistic and biographical approaches.[143] He suggests to work on cognitive restructuring by thinking about God, opening new experiences by exploring emotions and re-narrating the biography including the relationship to God. The basis for every pastoral care intervention should be solidarity with the depressed from a congregational network – and thus, pastoral care becomes the work of a whole congregation, not only the pastor.[144]

Some additional suggestions for pastoral care with depressed people are:

- *Religious and spiritual accompaniment*: The depressive person is also still a religious and spiritual person. In the mental health system, a pastoral care worker is the professional for religious questions. He can encourage the depressive person to raise questions about God, beliefs and emotions. He or she should be attentive to religious coping mechanisms and strengthen positive coping by allowing complaining and articulation of problems and at the same time also rely on spiritual and religious resources.[145] Some conversation techniques can also be supportive for ministers like motivational interviewing that tries to focus not only on burdensome aspects of life but rather tries to implement some change of view.[146]

141 Cf. Morgenthaler, *Seelsorge*, 190.

142 Cf. chapter II.1 in this volume: Annette Haußmann, Beate Jakob, and Birgit Weyel, *Depression and Pastoral Care from the Viewpoint of Pastors in Germany*. As well as Klessmann, "Pastoralpsychologische Seelsorge mit depressiven Menschen," 27–42, 28 and 42.

143 Cf. Klaus Depping, *Depressive alte Menschen seelsorgerlich begleiten. Auswege aus Schwermut und Verzweiflung* (Hannover: Lutherisches Verlagshaus, 2000).

144 Cf. Weyel and Jakob, "Kirchengemeinden als soziales Netz," 12–18. Also Klessmann, "Pastoralpsychologische Seelsorge mit depressiven Menschen," 27–42, 41 and Kunz, "Beten in der Anfechtung," 159–192. For a general approach of a pastoral care in the context of the church congregation cf. Wolfgang Drechsel, *Gemeindeseelsorge* (Leipzig: Evangelische Verlagsanstalt, 2nd ed. 2016)

145 A study has shown that positive religious coping can be supported by pastors. Cf. P. S. Bay, D. Beckman, J. Trippi, R. Gunderman and C. Terry, "The effect of pastoral care services on anxiety, depression, hope, religious coping, and religious problem solving styles: a randomized controlled study," *Journal of Religion and Health* 47(1) (2008): 57–69. Examples for approaching religious and spiritual resources can be found in: Heike Schneidereit-Mauth, *Ressourcenorientierte Seelsorge. Salutogenese als Modell für seelsorgerliches Handeln* (Gütersloh: Gütersloher Verlagshaus, 2015).

146 Cf. Annette Haußmann, "Wege zur Veränderung: Motivierende Gesprächsführung," in *Das Depressions-Buch für Pflege- und Gesundheitsberufe: Menschen mit Depressionen gekonnt pflegen und behandeln*, eds. Thomas Hax-Schoppenhorst and Stefan Jünger (Bern: Hogrefe, 2016): 269–281.

- *Using biblical examples*: Depression is a young illness, considering the term and classification itself.[147] The symptoms, however, were already described in the Bible. For depressed people it can be helpful, if they realize that even 'heroes' of the Bible struggled with God like Job, who suffered from exhaustion, like Elijah who questioned Gods actions in the Lamentations.[148] Texts and rituals, Eucharistic experience, singing and praying can encourage to keep up the dialogue with God or meet religious or spiritual needs.[149]
- *Discovering the image of God and its biographical roots*: Being encouraged to express anger and protest towards God can be helpful as a form of constructive lamentation. It also helps to express anger that is often hidden behind a depression because people in depression do not allow themselves to be angry and thus turn the anger against themselves. Thus, expressing angry feelings towards God, expressing the sorrow of being forgotten or alone can be a first step to come in contact with God again. Also, the image of God and its rooting in the individual's biography can be explored to figure out if there are underlying convictions that could be changed or at least questioned. Glendon Moriarty suggests to integrate the image of God to pastoral care by accessing and scrutinizing, and then carefully help to change it.[150]
- *Mentioning suicidality*: Depressive persons are often suicidal. Therefore, it is necessary to figure out if the person has suicidal ideas or has already thought about definite methods to end his or her life. Most people are afraid to mention suicidality directly, but for the people affected, it can be a relief to finally talk about their feelings and thoughts. It is also possible and sometimes necessary to offer support from within the health system including further contacts and accompaniment. If there seems to be self-endangerment for the person, there should be an immediate attempt

147 Cf. Alan Ehrenberg, *Das erschöpfte Selbst: Depression und Gesellschaft in der Gegenwart*, Frankfurter Beiträge zur Soziologie und Sozialphilosophie, Vol. 6 (Frankfurt/Main: Campus, 2004).

148 Cf. Beate Jakob, "Bibelarbeit zum Thema Depression," in *Menschen mit Depression. Orientierungen und Impulse für die Praxis in Kirchengemeinden*, eds. Birgit Weyel and Beate Jakob (Gütersloh: Gütersloher Verlagshaus, 2014): 128–139.

149 Cf. Klessmann, "Pastoralpsychologische Seelsorge mit depressiven Menschen," 27–42, 41.

150 Cf. Glendon Moriarty, *Pastoral Care of Depression: Helping clients heal their relationship with God* (New York: Routledge, 2006).

to convince this person to go to a psychiatric hospital or at best to organize a transfer or accompany him or her there.[151]

- *Respecting one's own boundaries*: Offering support to depressed persons sometimes can be exhausting and challenging. It helps to see one's own resources and burdens and then also accept the limitations to help and offer support. An inner distance is also advisable since depressive moods easily affect both interacting partners in a vicious circle of depressive communication.[152]
- *Religion, meaning, and health are ultimately inaccessible*: Religion – from a theological perspective – is not a resource that is always available or teachable. Therefore, it remains important to point out that religion is a gift from God, although there are approaches in psychotherapy as well to integrate spirituality and religion as resources. This is the reason why theology and psychology, pastoral care workers and psychotherapists need to work together in a multi-professional setting in institutions but also in an outpatient setting.[153]

A lot of depressive disorders are not treated with psychotherapy because they are not recognized as a mental health problem. Hence, basic knowledge about depression is crucial. Pastors and also volunteer workers can help lead to an early detection of the problem and thus help people to get treatment in an early stage of the illness or to prevent it.[154] On the other hand, this does not mean a minister has to act as a therapist or to make a diagnose. Rather, he or she can accompany a person, mention changes in behavior or emotions and thus facilitate the admission to the professional health system.[155] Therefore, it is also useful to be informed about different possibilities of psychotherapy and medical help, as well as having information about the specific and holistic context of

---

151 Cf. Annette Haußmann and Friedemann Bresch, "Seelsorgerliche Gesprächsführung mit depressiven Menschen," in *Menschen mit Depression*, eds. Birgit Weyel and Beate Jakob (Gütersloh: Gütersloher Verlagshaus, 2014): 179–194, 193–194.

152 Cf. Haußmann and Bresch, "Seelsorgerliche Gesprächsführung" 179–194. Also Daniel Hell, "Psychodynamik der Depression und Achtsamkeit," in *Dunkle Nacht' und Depression: Geistliche und psychische Krisen verstehen und unterscheiden*, eds. Regina Bäumer and Michael Plattig (Ostfildern: Grünewald, 2008): 10–21, 16–17.

153 Cf. Birthe Boettcher, "Spiritual Care and multiprofessional collaboration of professionals in pastoral care and psychotherapy in outpatient care," in *Spiritual Care* (2018): 377–385.

154 Cf. Morgenthaler, *Seelsorge*, 187.

155 Cf. also chapter II.1 in this volume: Annette Haußmann, Beate Jakob and Birgit Weyel, *Depression and Pastoral Care from the Viewpoint of Pastors in Germany*.

depression from a sociological and systemic point of view.[156] Various reasons can cause and maintain a depressive episode. Therefore, a biopsychosocial understanding of the illness can be helpful. As religion is a part of this complex interaction, it is also important to integrate the religious or spiritual perspective into pastoral guidance. Some pastors try to help quickly with information or suggestions to improve or change the individual's constitution. This impulse is understandable but in most cases it is better to first listen and figure out what the depressed person needs and wants. The professional background of a pastoral care worker is the religious system. He or she is able to understand and reflect about the individual religious orienting system of the person seeking help and at the same time have the rich religious and spiritual tradition of the Bible and Christian congregations in mind. Concerninig meaning-making the pastor is a professional and therefore can help to find new perspectives on meaning in a biographical context. As to religious beliefs, it can help to explore with the other, whether and how religion and spirituality are helpful and protective to them or if harmful aspects are predominant.

7 Conclusion

There is a dynamic and ambivalent relationship between religion and depression rooted in the individual's path, and biography, which also leads to the notion that faith itself develops with different experiences.[157] As a dark phase in life can happen to anyone, depression affects the spiritual and religious life, too. The intertwined relation leads to religion influencing depression and vice versa: depression darkens every sphere in life and thus affects religion and belief as well. Many studies have shown that symptoms can be a dark, distant, angry image of God and low self-esteem, religiously interpreted guilt and shame, suicidal ideas, and social problems within the religious community. On the other hand, positive effects from spirituality and religion can emerge and influence depression in a good way: buffering and preventing effects can be found in prayer and meditation, church attendance, forgiveness, and social support within a religious community and various other resources. Religion also offers a meaning system to the individual and its systemic context, thus it can provide a stabilizing orienting system. Depression is a treatable illness, and suffering from depressive symptoms

156 Cf. Morgenthaler, *Seelsorge*, 183–190.
157 Cf. Annette Haußmann, Ambivalenz und Dynamik. Religion in der häuslichen Pflege (Berlin: De Gruyter, 2019).

can be reduced with appropriate psychotherapy and sometimes medical treatment. Often, religious conflicts or problems disappear during treatment. Religion and spirituality should be addressed from a multi-professional perspective, integrating spiritual care, health professionals, and psychotherapists. Pastoral care especially can address spiritual or religious conflicts, provide rituals or guidance – particularly if depression is only sub-clinically relevant. But spirituality can be integrated into psychotherapy as well, if the patient's needs indicate an openness to this topic and the therapist is trained to do so.

II Studies

Annette Haußmann, Beate Jakob, and Birgit Weyel

Depression and Pastoral Care from the Viewpoint of Pastors in Germany

1 Introduction

Interestingly, very few studies have formerly dealt with pastoral care and the role of depression. But recently, some studies have pointed out that in dealing with mental diseases, church congregations can be helpful to those who suffer and their relatives. Pastors[1] often deal with depressed people in their professional practice, but mostly do not participate in a special training before doing so. In Germany, pastoral care is addressed during university education of pastors as well as during their practical training for the ministry in a more general sense (self-concept, role expectation, communication etc.), but not with a focus on mental health. Pastors, however, encounter the problem of mental diseases like depression in pastoral care situations such as grief, loss or illness. And depression can also play a role in everyday situations when pastoral care takes place more or less informally: Maybe at an event like a birthday visit to elderly pesons, or at a funeral, or after a Sunday service. Such situations are quite challenging for pastors as they normally do not have a specific training in dealing with mentally ill people. The specialization of healthcare chaplaincy in psychiatric clinics which is separated from pastoral care in congregations could be the cause for this lack of preparation. It is, however, possible to pursue further training in pastoral care[2] and appropriate special knowledge of mental disorders. But there is only a limited amount of special literature available to ministers that gives basic information about

1 The terms "pastor" and "minister" are terms used synonymously. Male and female pastors are both addressed with these terms.

2 Such courses in Clinical Pastoral Care (Klinische Seelsorge Ausbildung, KSA) are mainly offered by the German Association for Pastoral Psychology (Deutsche Gesellschaft für Pastoralpsychologie, DGfP). US studies also show that only a proportion of pastors received clinical pastoral education beforehand, cf. e.g. Michael Moran, Kevin J. Flannelly, Andrew J. Weaver, Jon A. Overvold, Winfried Hess and Jo Clare Wilson, "A study of pastoral care, referral, and consultation practices among clergy in four settings in the New York City area," *Pastoral Psychology* 53(3) (2005): 255–265; Jennifer Payne, "The influence of secular and theological education on pastors' depression intervention decisions," *Journal of Religion and Health* 53(5) (2014): 1398–1413.

https://doi.org/10.1515/9783110674217-005

depression and practical knowledge how to deal with it in a pastoral care context.[3] But information is available. The German Association for Depression trains multipliers like teachers, ministers, police officers, pharmacists, and nursing teachers about depression as an illness and provides information about detecting depressive symptoms and possibilities of treatment.[4]

From an international perspective, studies indicate that pastors play a crucial role in not only identifying depressed individuals but also helping them to get professional help or support with spiritual issues arising during depression. Depression is one of the most frequent and most severe mental diseases in a congregation as perceived by ministers.[5] Only a small percentage of those meeting the criteria for a major depression episode seek professional help. They would first prefer to seek help in their social environment because there is less stigma in seeking help from a pastor than seeing a psychotherapist straight away. This, of course, is highly dependent on the culture and environment. Whereas in a more secular context pastors are less likely to be asked for help with a psychological problem, in a more religious context like in the US people more frequently seek support from a minister.[6] An individual with depressive symptoms is less likely to

3 German literature for pastors and volunteers in pastoral care: Jochen Sautermeister and Tobias Skuban, eds., *Handbuch psychiatrisches Grundwissen für die Seelsorge* (Freiburg: Herder, 2018); Michael Klessmann, "Pastoralpsychologische Seelsorge mit depressiven Menschen," in *Pastoralpsychologische Perspektiven in der Seelsorge*, ed. Michael Klessmann (Göttingen: Vandenhoeck & Ruprecht, 2017): 27–42; Christoph Morgenthaler, "Verletzlichkeit, psychische Krisen und Erkrankungen – das Beispiel Depression," in *Seelsorge*, Lehrbuch Praktische Theologie Vol. 3, ed. Christoph Morgenthaler (Gütersloh: Gütersloher Verlagshaus, 2009): 183–190; Klaus Kießling, *Seelsorge bei Seelenfinsternis* (Freiburg: Herder, 2002). In conjunction with the attention for psychic trauma due to war and escape in pastoral care with refugees over the last years the regardfulness for special needs of people with mental illness has increased. Cf. for example Maike Schult, *"Ein Hauch von Ordnung". Traumaarbeit als Aufgabe der Seelsorge*, Arbeiten zur Praktischen Theologie, vol. 64 (Leipzig: Evangelische Verlagsanstalt, 2020). English literature for pastors cf. e.g. Binford W. Gilbert, *The Pastoral Care of Depression: A Guidebook* (New York: Routledge, 2014); Glendon Moriarty, *Pastoral Care of Depression: Helping clients heal their relationship with God* (Binghamton: Routledge, 2006); Jaco J. Hamman, "Down and can't get up again: Serious depression," in *The Church Leader's Counseling Resource Book: A Guide to Mental Health and Social Problems*, eds. Cynthia Franklin and Rowena Fong (Oxford: Oxford University Press, 2011): 154–163.

4 Cf. Bündnis gegen Depression, in URL: https://www.deutsche-depressionshilfe.de (last accessed on 1 April 2020).

5 Cf. Teresa L. Kramer, Dean Blevins, Terri L. Miller, Martha M. Phillips, Vanessa Davis and Billy Burris, "Ministers' perceptions of depression: A model to understand and improve care," *Journal of Religion and Health* 46(1) (2007): 123–139.

6 To seek help from members of the clergy is less stigmatizing in the US than approaching a therapist, cf. Ratonia C. Runnels and Mel Stauber, "Today's best pastoral care: Church-based

seek help directly than just indirectly referring to the symptoms in the context of other problems like social problems or loneliness. Often it is the pastor who becomes aware of a mental health issue, or family members who express their concern.[7] In dealing with depression, a large part of the ministers still feel less competent in addressing depression than in dealing with other problems like grief, anxiety, or death.[8] This explains why most of the clergy want to have further training about depression, as more than three-quarters of the participants in a US study stated.[9] Professional cooperation and support on a multi-professional level is therefore mandatory for most members of clergy: they do not only refer to other professions, but also assist the depressed to seek help offered by other professionals; they often know competent psychotherapists, doctors or institutions who can be approached for consultation or information.[10]

Studies have also shown that during depression, religion and meaning become an issue. Belief systems that were undoubted before can be shaken to the core. Depression can lead to fundamental questions about one's own life, God and God's will, and the meaning of life. Feelings and cognitions like fundamental doubt, guilt or hopelessness can arise and also affect religious beliefs.[11] Religion offers resources but can also be a burdening for downcast individuals. Thus, pastoral care is not merely about addressing depression as a medical condition and helping the suffering to find psychotherapeutic or medical care in the health system, but also about offering a possibility that goes beyond: a church congregation and pastoral care can offer support to many people, regardless if they themselves are religious or not.[12] Therefore pastors and their perception,

---

mental health and social programs," in *The Church Leader's Counseling Resource Book: A Guide to Mental Health and Social Problems*, eds. Cynthia Franklin and Rowena Fong (Oxford: Oxford University Press, 2011): 431–448.

7 Cf. Teresa L. Kramer et al., "Ministers' perceptions of depression: A model to understand and improve care," *Journal of Religion and Health* 46(1) (2007): 123–139.

8 Cf. Michael Moran et al., "A study of pastoral care, referral, and consultation practices among clergy in four settings in the New York City area," *Pastoral Psychology* 53(3) (2005): 255–266.

9 Cf. Payne, "The influence of secular and theological education," 1398–1413.

10 Cf. Kramer et al., "Ministers' perceptions of depression," 123–139.

11 Cf. Birgit Weyel and Annette Haußmann, "Spiritualität und Depressivität," in *Menschen mit Depression. Orientierungen und Impulse für die Praxis in Kirchengemeinden*, eds. Birgit Weyel and Beate Jakob (Gütersloh: Gütersloher Verlagshaus, 2014): 19–27.

12 Pastors report integrating a spiritual and psychological knowledge in pastoral care by helping to support the mental health system, cf. John L. Young, Ezra E. H. Griffith and David R. Williams, "The integral role of pastoral counseling by African-American clergy in community mental health," *Psychiatric Services* 54(5) (2003): 688–692. Also, the study of Kramer et al., "Ministers' perceptions of depression," 123–139 has shown, that most of the pastors

knowledge and dealing with depression are often gatekeepers for the support system congregations can offer.[13] Additionally, they could even provide prevention through information and lowering thresholds to the mental health system for those in a depressed mood, before they enter a severe depression episode.

In light of this perception, the Tübingen research team wanted to know more about the specific role of the pastors addressing the problem of depression or even trying to help those suffering from depression. How are pastors reacting to those kinds of challenges in their everyday work? Is depression or are seemingly depressed people even a topic they are dealing with? In order to address these questions, the research team carried out a study with its main interest being if and how pastors come into contact with the topic of depression and how they are addressing and coping with it. According to the fact that depression and mental disease is not a part of the typical pastoral care training, the team also wanted to know if pastors felt well enough informed about depression and, if not, if they wanted to receive further education or information. The focus on depression in the context of pastoral care is due to the fact that a lot of people still perceive depression as a problem they would rather not talk about because they are ashamed of it. Depression still is an issue of stigmatization. Thus, the team assumed that depression-related symptoms would be addressed rather in a private and sheltered environment like a face-to-face pastoral care situation.

2 Methods and Participants

This study was conducted in Tübingen, a city in Southern Germany, in 2013 and involved trained male and female pastors.[14] First, we conducted four qualitative interviews with pastors that show a range of different degrees of expert knowledge

---

also use faith-based interventions in pastoral care in addition to medical treatment of the health care system. For advanced contributions to congregation as a network in the perspective of a network-analysis cf. Felix Roleder and Birgit Weyel, *Vernetzte Kirchengemeinde. Persönliche Beziehungen, religiöse Kommunikation, kirchliche Geselligkeit und zivilgesellschaftliche Beteiligung. Analysen zur Gesamtnetzwerkerhebung der V. Kirchenmitgliedschaftsuntersuchung der EKD* (Leipzig: Evangelische Verlagsanstalt 2019).

13 Cf. Curtis J. VanderWaal, Edwin I. Hernandez and Alix R. Sandman, "The gatekeepers: Involvement of Christian clergy in referrals and collaboration with Christian social workers and other helping professionals," *Social Work and Christianity* 39(1) (2012): 27–51.

14 Birgit Weyel, Annette Haußmann, Beate Jakob and Stefanie Koch, *Menschen mit Depression: Orientierungen und Impulse für die Praxis in Kirchengemeinden* (Gütersloh: Gütersloher Verlagshaus, 2014).

about depression (I-2, I-3, I-5, I-13).[15] One pastor is an expert in clinical pastoral care and works in a psychiatric context. Therefore, he was expected to be the most experienced of the group in dealing with depression (I-13). Two of the interviewed pastors were already making depression their special subject in the congregation and thus had some experience in talking about it. We considered them to be some kind of pastoral care experts in the field of depression but also they have experienced the limitations of their knowledge considering the complexity of depression (I-2, I-3). Thirdly, we interviewed one pastor who had had no experience with depression so far (I-5).

After interviewing this group of pastors with a qualitative approach, we conducted a second quantitative study in one church district in the south of Germany.[16] All 71 pastors in this district with 45 church congregations were invited to participate and 27 of them answered the questionnaire about pastoral care and depression (38%). The mean age was 50.4 years (SD=6.10 years) and the majority was male (m=76.2%, f=23.8%). 90% of the pastors had a full-time position in a church congregation, 5% occupied a specialized pastoral care position and another 5% had a position with a special function (Table 1).

The questionnaire was completed online with a research tool (soscisurvey.de). The questions addressed the contexts of pastoral care (Where, when and how often does pastoral care with people in a depressed mood take place?), the important topics of those conversations and the emotions of the help seeking person, and finally a reflection on their pastoral care itself (How do the pastors evaluate themselves and perceive their own pastoral care practice? How would they like to be supported with trainings?). SPSS 19 was used to evaluate the data.

---

15 All interviews are archived and can be retrieved at the Chair of Practical Theology at Tübingen University. The questions were developed by the research team under the special direction of Birgit Weyel and conducted by research assistant Stefanie Koch in 2011 and 2012. Some excerpts from the interviews are have already been in: Stefanie Koch, "Wie können Kirchengemeinden depressiv kranke Menschen und ihre Angehörigen unterstützen? Interviews mit ausgewählten Personengruppen," in *Menschen mit Depression: Orientierungen und Impulse für die Praxis in Kirchengemeinden*, eds. Birgit Weyel and Beate Jakob (Gütersloh: Gütersloher Verlagshaus, 2014): 53–97.

16 A short overview of this study was published by Annette Haußmann, "Empirische Ergebnisse aus der Online-Umfrage unter Pfarrerinnen und Pfarrern," in *Menschen mit Depression: Orientierungen und Impulse für die Praxis in Kirchengemeinden*, eds. Birgit Weyel and Beate Jakob (Gütersloh: Gütersloher Verlagshaus, 2014): 45–52.

Table 1: Statistics of the Sample for the Quantitative Study.

Variable	Results
Age	Mean: 50.4 years SD: 6.10 years
Gender	76.2% male 23.8% female
Function in the church congregation	90% pastor in a church congregation 5% special pastoral care position 5% special other position
Type of employment	80% full-time 20% part-time

3 Results of the Study

In presenting the results of the study, qualitative and quantitative data will be mixed to complement each other. This ensures that quantitative data will be more transparent and qualitative data will be put into a broader framework. First, there is a summary of the contexts of pastoral care (3.1). Second, emotions and mood of the help-seeking persons will be shown (3.2). Third, contents of pastoral care conversations are presented (3.3). Finally, there is the reflection on the pastoral care practice (3.4). Please note that these results are always the perception of the pastors themselves. So, if we are talking about the mood of the depressed help-seekers, this is always the perception of the pastor, not the exact mental state of the depressed person. Furthermore, we speak about "depressed mood" rather than "depression", because the pastors usually have no clinical training and thus are not able to tell whether the symptoms really indicate a manifest depression. The term "depressed mood" is more open for a wide range of phenomena. Additionally, pastors often are among the first contact persons from whom people seek help and thus most people have not yet been diagnosed clinically.

3.1 Contexts of Pastoral Care and Depression

According to the survey, over a period of three months there are on the average seven conversations with people in a depressed mood. The variation is widespread between two and thirty conversations in such a time period. These types of conversations make up about 16% of all pastoral care situations, ranging between 4% and 80% of all conversations. About half of the participants estimate that the number of help-seeking depressed persons has been the same during the last few years, whereas 28% state that their numbers have even increased. The contexts of pastoral care in which the topic of depression plays a role or pastors encounter people in a depressed mood are diverse, too. Most of these conversations take place in acute crises. Surprisingly, a third of the pastors said that they also were confronted with depression in passing situations. This gives a strong sense that depression is something people often do not communicate directly, but pastors are sensing in everyday contact situations that something is wrong with the person they are talking to. On the other hand, this also gives insight into the sensitivity of ministers. Rarely, other staff members in the congregation, such as voluntary workers, teachers or nursery school teachers, are referring to the pastor with a certain pastoral care situation (Figure 1).

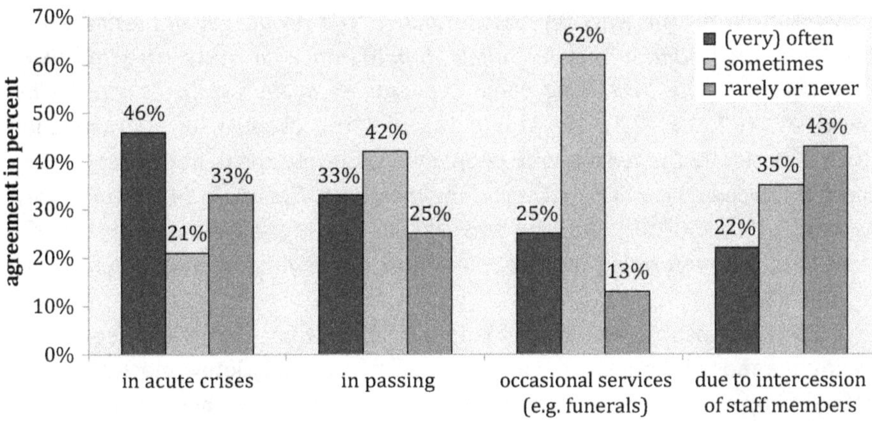

Figure 1: Occasions for pastoral care with people in a depressed mood. The 5-item-scale of agreement was summarized to 1+2 (very often and often), 3 sometimes, 4+5 (rarely and never).

Additionally, pastors point out that they often come across depression during birthday visits to older people, or anniversaries. In the private environment of their home, these people tend to open up to the minister and talk about their sorrows and problems. Most of these contacts were known to the pastor beforehand; 52% say that this is the case often or very often. It was rather rare that the pastor did not know the person from the church congregation: when they were unknown it was either because they belonged to other parishes (33% agreed to "rarely") or because they were distant to church (30% agree to "rarely"). This underlines that the congregation is an important place for those who are in need of help, and most of them are members of the congregation who already are in close contact with the pastor. It is important to keep in mind that congregational pastoral care covers a variety of encounters. Exactly this openness to situations for pastoral care – or not – is not exclusive, but specific for congregations.[17]

The qualitative results also indicate that pastors are confronted with those in a depressed mood in a variety of situations. A pastor describes these occasions: "*All those [situations], I face in my daily work. That can be during conversations before a funeral of course, but it can also be the case at conversations before a baptism or when meeting with the parents of confirmands or in all generations, also meetings with elderly people. So, it can concern every generation*" (I-5, 32–36). Depression thus is not only present in a minster's daily work experience, and also not limited to a certain group or age. However, certain groups are more present in a minister's work than others – for example, as mentioned above, the birthday visit to older people.[18] Another pastor points to cases where he meets other people with depressed moods: "*Old people whom I visit for their birthday in their homes. They live alone, family rather far away. They're talking about tiredness, they're talking about the badness of the world. They're feeling downcast.*" (I-2, 205–211). He also points out the problem of stigmatization which is basically the reason why people would rarely speak about depression: "*But it is concealed very very strongly, smothered up. Especially in a rural context like here.*" (I-2, 160–161). And he adds: "*They say my self-concept is that of a strong and top-performing human being. And this is fundamentally dominant.*" (I-2, 168–169).

Only a few people would speak openly about their depressive feelings or already diagnosed depression. Often, the pastors already knew most of the depressed people. I-2 talks about three people with depressed mood he often is in

17 "It has become clear that forms of encounters of pastoral care in a congregational setting are extremely manifold. Only the synopsis of its opportunities presents [...] a concrete-related approach to an answer of the context related question: 'What is pastoral care in a congregation?'" (Wolfgang Drechsel, *Gemeindeseelsorge* [Leipzig: Evangelische Verlagsanstalt, 2015], 76) (Ger.: Es ist deutlich geworden, dass die seelsorglichen Begegnungsformen in der Gemeinde äußerst vielfältig sind. Erst die Zusammenschau ihrer Möglichkeit präsentiert [...] einen konkretionsbezogenen Zugang zu einer Antwort auf die kontextbezogene Frage: Was ist Seelsorge in der Gemeinde?")

18 Cf. In the perspective of everyday spiritual care (Alltagsseelsorge), the analysis of communication on the occasion of a birthday visit: Eberhard Hauschildt, *Alltagsseelsorge. Eine sozio-linguistische Analyse des pastoralen Geburtstagsbesuches* (Göttingen: Vandenhoeck & Ruprecht 1996).

contact with: "*This woman from [name of town], I have visited her a few times. The classic birthday visit. [...] I visited her in the nursing home and she told me the depression came over night, as a sort of illness.*" (I-2, 24–29). Some of those people are also seeking new possibilities to meet others in a congregation if they are in a phase free of symptoms. I-2 talks about an encounter with a female person that was new in their congregation: "*[She] entered the church, she had a stable phase at this moment. A person that recently moved into town. That was a good meeting, a nice meeting. She could openly talk about her depression.*" (I-2, 44–47). He also mentioned the birthday phone call he made and did not reach her. He then met her on the street a few weeks later and talked to her. At that point, she was experiencing a depressive episode: "*I then met her briefly on the street and spoke to her and she just said that she was badly off.*" (I-2, 51–52). This short episode also shows that it is the pastor who is aware of the problem of depression, especially when he or she knows about the illness, and reaches out to the person and shows interest in her situation. The minister mentioned as well that it makes a big difference if the person in need is embedded in the context of the congregation. One of the depressed people volunteers in a Bible study group in the congregation and participates even if she is in a depressive episode. The pastor notices her just being quiet and rarely talking, just sitting there, and sometimes leaving at the end of the group sessions without saying anything, but then he just leaves her alone because he knows about her condition.

Another pastor also points out that it is during Sunday service that he encounters people with a depressed mood: "*One thinks many things, one senses many things if one is holding a Sunday service. If you are standing on the pulpit, you can sense that there are humans with a depressed mood. I don't want to say straight away that they are suffering from depression, but they are downhearted.*" (I-3, 19–22). When preparing the service, he thinks about those who are especially in need of a good word in their life: "*One always has some people in mind ... but ultimately this is just an assumption. One thinks: That would be the right word for him or her. [Interviewer (=I): Mhm.] Yes, I think, that for sure I'm encountering humans without knowing for sure if they have a depression or not.*" (I-3, 31–36). This pastor also has a strong feeling for the mental state of those who are participating in the service and elsewhere. He also leads a group for mentally ill people which makes him aware of the different mental problems in his daily work. He also mentioned occasions like birthdays: "*And on birthday visits I realize: Depression due to loneliness. One quickly realizes that. So to speak, the human being that is just with himself for the whole day, and perhaps with his cat, if he's lucky. Therefore, loneliness [I: Yes.] makes depressive. Where the challenge would be to establish social contacts somehow.*" (I-3, 103–108). This also points out that professional experience plays a crucial role for pastors being alert to the phenomenon of depression. One pastor explains about this development of professional sensitivity: "*I became more sensitive over the years. For instance, if people are very plaintive, if they're, uhm, saying a lot of negative things all the time. Or if nothing is right for them, and the world simply is always sombre. Uhm, as a young man, I just thought: Well, this is just a pessimist. But I have tried to listen more carefully*" (I-13, 172–177).

It is, however, often the pastor's own awareness for the situation and his sensitivity for the people he encounters that results in a specific pastoral care situation like a conversation, a sermon, a group meeting or even a long-term accompaniment.

3.2 Issues, Mood, and Emotions of Depressed People in Pastoral Care

Mostly women are perceived to be depressed in a congregational environment. 65% of the participating ministers said that more females with depression related symptoms are looking for support in pastoral care. Also, mostly older people are the recipients of pastoral care, as 73% of the pastor's state that they are often or very often talking to this group of elderly people. This might be due to the demographic structure of many congregations: women as well as older people are over-represented in church congregations. Different from the statement of the pastor (I-5) who pointed out that depression occurs in every generation, the quantitative study reports that only 6.7% of the pastors say they are often in contact with teenagers or young adults in a depressive mood (16 to 30 years), whereas 53% rarely or never and 40% sometimes meet with depressed persons within this group of age. Half of the pastors (42%) have to do often or very often with middle-aged depressed people (31 to 60 years), the other half sometimes (48%). This clearly points out that young people with depression are rather not perceived to be depressed or they are simply underrepresented in pastors' daily work experience.

A closer look at the specific emotions and topics to be addressed in pastoral care situations shows that ministers are mostly perceiving thoughts or feelings of hopelessness, feelings of inferiority and a dark view of themselves. Quite rarely, problems with medication or social isolation are articulated in pastoral care. Suicidal thoughts, however, are mentioned relatively often. On the average such thoughts are mentioned 1.5 times in three months, variating between 1 and 5 times. This is quite often, considering that such contacts with people in a depressed mood only occur on an average of seven times per quarter. It is also quite striking when we consider that such thoughts and feelings are often interpreted because they are hidden or concealed in other conversation topics.

Pastors noticed such implicit suicidal ideas as often as open conversation about someone's suicidality. On the other hand, suicidal ideas are not only hidden, but pastors also feel that their intervention is sometimes too late. One interviewee had held some funerals after suicides, but he added the impression that the depressed person did not want to talk to him about suicidal ideas: "*I had no one saying that he or she was calling for help [I: Mhm.] And so, as I already pointed out, that problem I felt with all three depressed people, that they shut themselves off like I had the impression I couldn't reach out to them even if I wanted to.*" (I-2, 253–258). This behavior is, so he explains, due to depression and the impossibility of opening up to others. Similarly, one pastor said he was not aware of thoughts of suicide: "*I think it has to do a lot with being ashamed, that this human wouldn't dare to speak about it. So, uhm, I, for me, I can't make out any case where I did know with that beforehand.*" (I-3, 117–121). Also, there is the notion of suicide or suicidal ideas being very shameful to religious people, especially the older generation. Accordingly, one pastor says this also has to do with the Christian tradition: "*And that that is mentioned still today, that this [suicide] is a cardinal sin, and it also is a chapter of church history, we still have to deal with and process today.*" (I-13, 220–222). In his view, older religious people would rather say something like: "*Minister, I have done something really stupid – and then I immediately knew*" (I-13, 216). This once more clarifies that it is again the pastor and his awareness for a phenomenon of suicidal ideas and thoughts of suicide and that he is able to speak about this. Similarly, pastor 5 clarifies that he would speak about that topic very clearly: "*That occurs, that is expressed. I already said, adults as well as … really, I, I, I would be very open about this, offensively, especially concerning children.*" (I-4, 63–65).

Clearly, the mood of the suffering person could also very strongly affect the minister's mood as well, so it is difficult for him to deal with the depressed. Pastor 2 shows how strongly he could feel the darkness of the depression pulling him down. "*It is a night ride. A night ride that cannot be compared with anything. That won't lead back into the light. That is the point. In many pastoral conversations you can really dig deep with them, but they want to go back into the light again.*" (I-2, 432–435). He says that with depressed people this is not possible anymore. "*This experience I haven't had yet [with the depressed]. And that is why I would hesitate to go into that labyrinth with them without knowing how to get out of there again.*" (I-2, 437–439). This statement clarifies how difficult it is for a minister to not only deal with the depressed person, saying appropriate things, but also to keep in mind his own resources and limitations in order to protect his own psyche from being affected too strongly the interviewee spoke of dark emotions in the metaphor of a "labyrinth" that makes it hard to find a way back out.

3.3 Content of Pastoral Care Conversation: Religion as a Topic?

Pastoral care is also an occasion to talk about religious struggles like doubts or questions, whether God has abandoned a person or punished her or him with this illness of depression. Such issues concerning the belief system of religious individuals are quite often mentioned. About half of the ministers (48%) perceived explicitly religious topics to be mentioned sometimes, but 42% said that those issues were a subject of discussion often or very often. Indicating that such issues are important in pastoral care and being mentioned in most of the conversations, we also wanted to know what problems concerning faith were mentioned exactly.

Religious doubts and feelings about being abandoned by God are most often emerging in pastoral care conversations. 71% of the pastors perceive them to occur often or very often. Secondly, feelings of guilt are the topic (29% very often and often, 47% sometimes). Over half of the pastors report about people in a depressed mood that are afraid of a punishing or threating God (56% sometimes). Figure 2 also shows that depression strongly affects the thoughts and feelings about faith and God and thus pastoral care is an important place to discuss such issues. Additionally, some pastors mentioned theodicy or problems in social relationships affected by change of the belief system to be of importance in conversations. According to the participants of the quantitative study, a depressive mood also leads to problems in religious practice because people cannot participate in church activities like Sunday services or group gatherings.

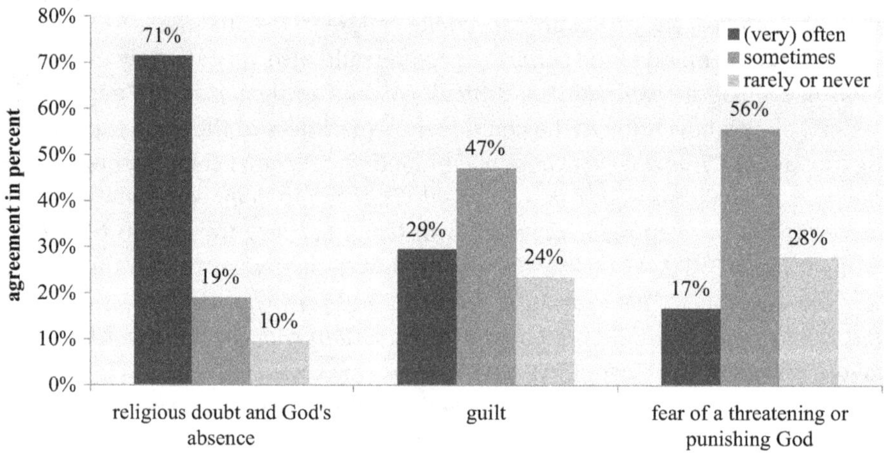

Figure 2: Religious topics and feelings in pastoral care: "How often are such topics articulated in pastoral care?" The 5-item-scale of agreement was summarized to 1+2 (very often and often), 3 sometimes, 4+5 (rarely and never).

The individual's understanding of religion plays an important role: "*Well, one says God. Another one says: community, church*" (I-2, 478). The qualitative results underline the presence of topics like theodicy and doubt. Some are asking God: "*Why is God letting this happen, why am I always having such a hard time?*" (I-3, 325–226). So, in the pastor's opinion the individual's religious framework with its beliefs, feelings and behavior is crucial for the way of dealing with the problem of a depressive mood. Also, the qualitative interviews showed how faith is strongly affected by depression. One pastor points out that there are two different ways of how religion plays a role in his conversations. On one hand, he links depression to a strict religious background: "*There are people with a very pious background, and after their second sentence it is obvious how many feelings of guilt there are because they have a totally wrong impression of piety and are influenced by religion in a way that can only make them ill, yes. And it is also clear how much burden they bear all the time and how little real liberation through Jesus there is.*" (I-5, 424–428). He also talks about a lack of honesty in a highly religious environment: "*I am experiencing a lot of lies. Many many lies, especially in a pious area, in a Christian environment. And, uhm, I think this is the point that depression has to do a lot with lies, with self-deception. Uhm, and that is according to our culture of parishes that demands such lies of people: you have to show that you are very pious.*" (I-5, 358–363). On the other hand, there are those with a lack of orientation in life: "*But there is also the other, the other direction. That individuals uhm uhm are empty, an inner emptiness in their life, yes, they never experienced or learned about faith or religion, and they are clearly experiencing deficits. Also of a basic comfort or of meaning, of orientation*" (I-5, 430–434). Concerning the feeling of guilt, for religious individuals there is the experience of feeling guilty because they are people without energy and therefore are not able to sort out their everyday life: "*one can't cook anymore, one can't care for the kids anymore, one fails at the job and so on*" (I-13, 67–68). And there is a religious side to this feeling of guilt as well: "*I have encountered often, that uhm, God is receding into far distance. And this is what is experienced as tremendously agonizing, especially for very religious, faithful people. They say, I'm praying, but it feels like a wall. So, I'm talking, like against a wall. God is not tangible anymore for me, not sensible, not perceptible anymore. And uhm … this loss of God's closeness or the perceived distance of God, one can elevate this theologically and say, the perceived hell, some even experience it as hell.*" (I-13, 70–76). Thus it is important to notice that during depression, faith also is strongly affected by the loss of feelings, emptiness or loss of energy.

But interestingly, pastors also point out the constructive role religion can play during depression and the needs people with a depressive mood are expressing: They long "*for a power that can accomplish what no man can accomplish. Namely, really a light, so to speak, that cuts through the dark and brings warmth and protection in which such a person who has the feeling of constantly falling and being isolated can feel safe and relevant. That is what religion is for.*" (I-2, 481–488). This longing for a light is also understood as a metaphor for his own experiences in dealing with depressed people (see 3.4). Some individuals also find support in religious beliefs during their depressive episodes. One person said to a pastor: "*I know these valleys of depression [I: Mhm.] I know, in this moment I'm feeling left alone, but I already know that. But I also know, coming from Psalm 23, that this sinister valley will be over some day. [I: Mhm.] And I'll have to wait until that moment comes. But I would never have the idea to lament before God.*" (I-3, 336–344). This minister also senses that religion plays a role during pastoral care conversations, at least in a nonverbal sense. "*So, obviously I'm representing something at least. Well, God is always there, but, he is not coming into the house with me, but obviously something is going on at this very moment, where they could sense: oh, maybe there actually is something like a hold.*" (I-3, 259–264), and he adds: "*In the very moment of the pastor's presence, God is somehow present, too.*" (I-3, 280–281). This leads to the question, how the minsters themselves deal with the pastoral care situation with depressed or downcast individuals.

3.4 Reflections on Pastoral Care Practice: How do Pastors Deal with Depression?

It has already been mentioned how difficult it is for pastors to react to people's depressive, specific mood, behavior, and feelings. They also affect the ministers themselves (see 3.2). Often pastors are feeling overwhelmed when they first have to deal with people in a depressed mood. Dealing with depressed individuals is challenging, as one of them reflects: "*Today I think I made the typical beginners' mistakes in pastoral care. That you try, so to speak, to turn a depressed human towards the sun. But that was pure pure self-protection, I think that today.*" (I-2, 30–33). The experience of depression mainly makes the pastors feel helpless and insecure. Pastor 2 tries to react with methods he knows from his pastoral care education and training: "*Therefore, I am reacting with the tools they taught us, the possibilities of intervention and of pastoral care and Rogers*[19] *and all that fuss, but*

19 The interviewee refers to Carl Rogers (1902–1987) with his person-centered approach to understanding personality and human relationships. His work found wide acceptance and his concept of interpersonal communication is a basic tool in the pastoral counselling

I already told you, that I feel rather helpless, that is almost a sort of self-defence to not be dominated by that emotion so strongly." (I-2, 385–390). But clearly, this seems not to work because the usual methods and rules of conversation don't seem to be working with depressed people. And additionally, his desire to help and act is pulling him down because his attempts to do so ultimately fail. So, this pastor feels more like he tries, but does not succeed in dealing with the illness or affected mood. When asked about how he is shaping pastoral care for humans in a depressed mood, he answers: "*I don't do that. Because that would mean that I could deal constructively with this topic. And that requires something I don't have: real competence. Therefore it is rather a reacting than an acting.*" (I-2, 375–379). He also tries to respect and care for his own limits by maintaining contact with the depressed person, but by also not expecting too much of his ability to help: "*I noticed [. . .] that I am glad when I notice, or when I know that I can protect myself a little, that I perceive the condition as it is, and that I try to bear it as best as I can. That means if I called the woman again for her birthday, I asked, how are you doing?, [says] I'm not doing well. Mhm. The medication doesn't work? No, they don't work. Mhm. Then I congratulate her on her birthday, and I will pray for you. Thank you. Goodbye. Like that.*" (I2, 443–453) Nevertheless, despite his reflected dealing with depression and his thoughtful perception of the situation, he is left with the feeling of struggling with his professional ideals: "*You cannot shine with that. You cannot shine with that. But I really didn't know then, I really didn't have an idea what else.*" (455–458).

Most of the pastors are also seeking help from other professionals when encountering or suspecting a problem of depression. 71% of the ministers in the quantitative study are giving pastoral care support themselves, but at the same time point out the importance to get professional medical care. On the contrary, only 5% keep the contact short because they are in contact with professional mental health care like a doctor or psychiatrist. 24% of the respondents state that in most cases a longer or long-term accompaniment is established with the help-seeking person. Also, 75% of the respondents are in contact with doctors, psychotherapists or advisory services whom they can contact in the case of emergency. Thus, a strong network and support system seems to be available for the pastors, and it is utilized at least in difficult situations. The majority of the pastors are able to identify the symptoms of a depression correctly, but still

training (clinical-pastoral training). Cf. Carl R. Rogers, Therapeut und Klient. Grundlagen der Gesprächspsychotherapie (München: Kindler, 1977).

38% are uncertain. This indicates a need for more psychological and medical information. Furthermore, we asked if the pastors wanted more information or training concerning depression. Only 33% felt well informed about the illness, whereas 43% felt more or less informed and only 24% felt well prepared.

These data show that there is a need for training and information concerning depression. More than two-thirds of the pastors wish to have further training and information about depression whereas only a third feels well prepared for pastoral care with depressive individuals. All in all, many pastors are pointing out they want to provide better support to people in a depressive mood and their relatives, but they would need better training to give adequate help. These results indicate a need for training courses linking psychology and theology, perhaps also combining tools of pastoral care and psychotherapy. For example, Pastor 2, who already made depression a special topic in his congregation, is refining this issue of bridging the psychological knowledge about depression and theology:

"*We are having the chance, as the only ones, not just to give others various information on a factual level, but also to transcend this level to a level of meaning. Especially, when we are linking Christian tradition, dogmatics, pastoral care, … just theology with this experience. That means that two things are happening. On the one hand, informational knowledge, so to speak, is getting refined through this level of meaning. On the other hand, it is also the talking about God and theology that is getting sharpened, it is that simple.*" (I-2, 529–536).

Digging deeper into pastoral care from a practical viewpoint, a closer look to the qualitative results shows that there are indeed different ways of dealing with depressive moods. Pastor 3 states that he feels that "*those humans need a lot of listening*" (I-3, 214) and he is willing to give them such attention: "*I am there! That people are feeling, at least temporarily, […] I am there and completely there for them.*" (I-3, 230–233). But he also draws a clear limit: "*And I'm realizing that I have to be careful with myself. Because they need me very, very urgently and they pull strongly. [I: Mhm.] And it is hard to reflect to them, that uhm … there's a limit, that not everyone is able to give as much as they would need now.*" (I-3, 81–85). He is therefore signalling: "*I am going with you up to a certain limit, but when I'm there, I'm there for you completely.*" (I-3, 235–236). To give unconditional attention is one way to deal with people in a depressed mood. Like Pastor 3, another one sees his role in giving such special acknowledgement: "*It is the small things, where humans are sensing and experiencing: Wow, there's someone that sees me! And, uhm, I think that is the minimum factor in our society, to experience at all that I'm someone to be seen as the one I really am. And not again to be seen as someone who the others want him to be, to be like that or to will be like that.*" (I-5, 92–96).

Others are trying to get a hold on information or tools themselves. Since there are no professional trainings, they look for appropriate literature or talk to other professionals. One pastor is talking a lot to his wife who is a systemic therapist. Another minister searched for literature, but could not find comprehensive, professional books: "*What I know about the medical aspects? Not a lot. I don't know a lot. And that means, that this is a request to our pastoral care education, because we haven't heard anything about that. Otherwise, I have to say that the uhm literature is miserable. [...] Theologians mainly tried in their books to be the better doctors.*" (I-2, 337–341). All in all, it is safe to say that pastors perceive a lack of good information and training about depression in pastoral care.

Religion can be an important resource not only for the individuals in a depressed mood, but also for the pastors and pastoral care itself. When asked about the understanding of pastoral care, a remarkable number of respondents stated that they would also pray in a pastoral care context (14% fully agreed, 19% rather agreed). Religion is also something to rely on as a basis in spiritual counselling, like one minister, quoting John 8, 32, points out: "*It is the Holy Spirit, who, as a spirit of truth, leads us into freedom. And, uhm, and there's a power behind that, which is just more than the notion of therapeutic pastoral care, thus, that is just the thing, yes. The truth will make you free, they say, and that is also true in a secular context. That is also valid in a therapeutic context. But as Christians we are coming from a different source of power.*" (I-5, 385–391). This kind of power also helps the pastor to ?? Also, another one commented on the importance of the biblical tradition: "*If you take a closer look at the Christian tradition, and the biblical tradition, too, then you realize that people had to do with depression throughout the centuries, starting with the biblical ages, and they have left a testimony. And this experience of depression also found its way into the literature of the Bible, and into spiritual scriptures as well. And therefore, you can also draw from this treasure of experiences, from those agonizing experiences, too, of course, as a pastoral carer.*" (I-13, 45–52). To support the depressed individual, he uses a variety of prayers or biblical phrases. In the Psalms and Lamentations, he finds many appropriate examples to express feelings of despair, loss of energy or even the absence of God. There is also the structure, as he argues, of lamentation turning into joy and vitality again which makes it easier to talk about the possibility of dynamics and change. He also found it helpful to tell stories of the Bible (e.g. Elijah in the desert, I Kings 19). According to the loss of faith during episodes without hope or in a depressed mood, he also tries to hold on to hope for the depressed person, as a kind of agency: "*To hope for the depressed person, who isn't able to do this anymore. Uhm, to say, the doctor can tell, in my experience, every depressive episode comes to an end finally. And it will be better again, uhm. But as a pastoral carer one can say as well, yes, I do believe firmly that you, that you as well, will again feel the closeness of God. This will change again.*" (I-13, 86–90). He even offers to pray for the depressed and acts before God on behalf of those, who do not feel the presence of God anymore. One can, however, not say for sure whether this helps the depressed or rather the pastor himself, who tries to cling on to hope and tries not to be hopeless because he perceives this to be his job during the accompaniment of the depressed. However, it is important to note that most of the pastors in the study struggle very intensely with the gap between wanting to help people with a depressed mood on the one hand, and their possibilities, methods, and resources in pastoral care on the other hand. But after all it is more important that the pastors are aware of depression in a congregational context and reflect on it and on including possible ways of improvement in education and professional collaboration.

4 Summary and Consequences

The results of our limited study cannot be generalized because they only give material about one church district in Southern Germany. Still, it is the first study to address the issue of depression in the context of pastoral care. The results have shown clearly that there is a lot of interest to help those in a depressed mood, but that there is also a variety of issues, feelings, and problems pastors encounter when trying to give support. The contexts where pastors, meet with people in a depressive mood are various and it strongly depends on the pastors' own knowledge and awareness about depression as a phenomenon if and how often they come across such situations. Another important observation is that not only older people, but also younger ones and middle-aged people can be affected by depression: a pastor might overestimate the number of older ones because he is meeting them more often in his daily routine or when younger people are depressed their mood might manifest differently and remain unnoticed.

In the perception of the respondents, religious topics, especially doubt and distance to God, often occur. Not only for religious individuals, but also for those who are looking for orientation, meaning, and guidance in life, religious questions and issues are something a pastor might be asked about or addressed. Therefore, it seems to be important to recognize such topics as a secondary effect that comes with a depressed mood. Also, the religious context of the congregation as well as cultural imprint affects the way people talk and think about depression as an illness and deal with it differently. But the study also shows how important religion can be as a resource for the depressed and the pastors as well. Especially biblical and religious traditions were mentioned often by the pastors and were used during conversations. Also, praying could be a way to express feelings in a particular situation, but it has become apparent that humans in a depressive episode cannot easily pray or attend Sunday service, and this has to be taken into account carefully. It is important to make clear that medical treatment and psychological attendance do not supersede pastoral care because there are specific religious issues which are preferably to be addressed by a theological expert.

Dealing with depressed people is difficult and sometimes overwhelming as they tend to pull down the pastors' mood and they sometimes even seem to ask for more support than a pastor is able to give. Since pastors themselves are often under stress and the risk of burnout or depression is also an issue for them, they need to be aware of the limitations of their ability to support, and they also need supervision when caring for people with depression.[20] But on the other hand, depressed people who hesitate to seek professional help are threatened by loneliness

---

20 For burnout and depression among pastors cf. Laura K. Barnard and John F. Curry, "The Relationship of Clergy Burnout to Self-Compassion and Other Personality Dimensions," *Pastoral Psychology* 61(2) (2012): 149–163; Candace Coppinger Pickett, Justin L. Barrett, Cynthia B. Eriksson and Christina Kabiri, "Social Networks among Ministry Relationships: Relational Capacity, Burnout, & Ministry Effectiveness," *Journal of Psychology and Theology* 45 (2) (2017): 92–105; Noel Due and Kirsten Due, "Courage and comfort for pastors in need," *Lutheran Theological Journal* 52(3) (2018): 128–140; for German context cf. Arndt Büssing, Jochen Sautermeister, Eckhard Frick and Klaus Baumann, "Reactions and Strategies of German Catholic Priests to Cope with Phases of Spiritual Dryness," *Journal of Religion and Health* 56 (2017): 1018–1031; Eckhard Frick, Klaus Baumann, Arndt Büssing, Christoph Jacobs and Jochen Sautermeister, "Spirituelle Trockenheit – Krise oder Chance? Am Beispiel der römisch-katholischen Priesterausbildung," *Wege zum Menschen* 70(1) (2018): 61–77; Arndt Büssing, Federico Baiocco and Klaus Baumann, "Spiritual Dryness in Catholic Laypersons Working as Volunteers is Related to Reduced Life Satisfaction Rather than to Indicators of Spirituality," *Pastoral Psychology*, 67(1) (2018): 1–15; Andreas von der Heyl, *Zwischen Burnout und spiritueller Erneuerung. Studien zum Beruf des evangelischen Pfarrers und der evangelischen Pfarrerin* (Frankfurt am Main: Lang, 2003). Cf. also the excellent study of Iris Kuttler, *Pfarrer in der Krise? Zusammenhänge zwischen Arbeitsanforderungen im Pfarrberuf und dem Burnout-Syndrom* (Konstanz 2007), in URL: https://d-nb.info/1080879579/34 (last accessed on 1 April 2020); Friedrich Weber and Michael Strauß, "Burnout–Herausforderung für die Kirche," in *Die auszehrende Organisation*, eds. Dietrich von der Oelsnitz, Frank Schirmer and Kerstin Wüstner (Wiesbaden: Springer Gabler, 2014): 269–274; Judith Winkelmann, "Wie viel von 75% ist unendlich? Strukturelle Faktoren für Burnout als Herausforderung für die Supervision," *Pastoraltheologie* 100(4) (2011): 198–214; Judith Winkelmann, "Weil wir nicht vollkommen sein müssen." Zum Umgang mit Belastungen im Pfarrberuf (Stuttgart: Kohlhammer, 2019).

and isolation.[21] Thus, it is important to be able to count on the congregation as a whole community and to help those in a depressed mood to find professional help. Specific training and appropriate information is needed in congregations and for pastors to be prepared for this task.[22] Not only information and tools how to deal with depressive people, but also methods of self-protection and self-care should be integrated. If we are able to strengthen the competence of pastoral caregivers, this could not only lead to an improvement in pastoral care practice, but also help to reduce stigmatization and to be more open in dealing with the illness of depression.

21 Annette Haußmann, "Einsamkeit und Spiritualität," in *Das Einsamkeitsbuch. Wie Gesundheitsberufe einsame Menschen verstehen, unterstützen und integrieren können*, ed. Thomas Hax-Schoppenhorst (Bern: Hogrefe, 2018): 153–163.

22 Cf. Annette Haußmann, "Suche nach Spiritualität und Sinn bei Depression. Was können Seelsorge und Kognitive Verhaltenstherapie voneinander lernen?" in Spiritualität und Sinn. Seelsorge und Kognitive Verhaltenstherapie im Dialog, ed. Annette Haußmann and Rainer Höfelschweiger, (Leipzig: Evangelische Verlagsanstalt, 2020) (in press).

Birgit Weyel

What Motivates Volunteers in Congregations to Take Care of People with Mental Disorders?

Looking at Pastoral Counselling Provided by Volunteers in Local Congregations

1 Introduction

The commitment of volunteers is an important object of research because of the huge impact of volunteers' work in civil societies. Every five years since 1999, the so-called 'Der Deutsche Freiwilligensurvey' (German Volunteer Study) generates data about developments and trends in volunteer work in Germany, enabling political actors to draw consequences.[1] Both research on volunteer work and research on pastoral counselling have largely ignored counselling provided by volunteers in local congregations. However, this work is a very interesting part of voluntary services that contribute to the health resources of local congregations. While public preaching and the administration of sacraments are restricted to ordained ministers, pastoral counselling is a task open to every Christian and has a long-standing biblical tradition.[2] In poimenics, however, pastoral counselling by volunteers has only recently begun to be looked into.[3] Reasons for this delay are the strong professionalism and specialization of pastoral care. Consequently, Eberhard Hauschildt rightfully demanded that pastoral counselling by lay people should be an integral part of poimenics. The qualitative study of pastoral care resources in local congregations which is the basis of this chapter, tries to contribute to this goal.

1 Cf. Julia Simonson, Claudia Vogel and Clemens Tesch-Römer, eds., *Freiwilliges Engagement in Deutschland. Der Deutsche Freiwilligensurvey 2014* (Berlin: Springer-Verlag, 2017).

2 The theological concept of the Protestant church draws on the idea of the priesthood of all believers as can be found in the theological work of Martin Luther: *An den Christlichen Adel* (1520).

3 Cf. Jochen Schlenker, "Zur Sprache bringen. Supervision mit Ehrenamtlichen in der Ausbildung zur Seelsorgerin, zum Seelsorger," *WzM* 66 (2014): 273–288. Schlenker gives an overview of literature concerning volunteer work published in recent years. As an example of case studies with volunteers in the field of pastoral care among immigrants cf. Birgit Weyel, "Christian Communities in the Face of Immigration. Interreligious pastoral care among immigrants," *Salesianum 81* (2019): 216–232.

https://doi.org/10.1515/9783110674217-006

Considering the number of affected people in the overall population, also members of local congregations are affected by mental stress and mental disorders. One can even argue that a disproportionate number of people with mental disorders can be found in local congregations. This is due to the number of older people present in local congregations, the spiritual longing for healing that might be connected with the symptoms of exhaustion and meaninglessness, and the easy accessibility to activities (like grieving groups, etc.). These offerings can serve as a first step towards help for affected people and can complement public health services if these are well connected with a particular congregation.

Local congregations already serve as health resources: the social network dimension of local congregations – the opportunity to get to know people and to cultivate friendships – is equally true for other groups, clubs and associations. But local congregations especially offer opportunities to meet pastors, other church members, staff, and ill people and their relatives. For people with mental disorders, local churches can be important social places. This study argues that local congregations can make an essential contribution to mental health, offering social networks and places to interpret[4] illness and health, healing and salvation and the relation to the divine.

In this chapter we will present some results of a qualitative study in the field of spiritual care, which was conducted from 2010 to 2012 (Pilot-Project) and 2014 to 2015 (follow up) as part of the Modellprojekt Seelsorge. The main questions of the study are: What motivates volunteers in congregations to take care of people with mental disorders? What are their experiences? How do they reflect on their work in terms of their own self-concept? How do they describe their part in spiritual care? How do they evaluate their skills in the field? Where do they see their limitations and their relationship to professional health caregivers. With the qualitative approach, we can reconstruct their self-understanding by using their own words.

It is important to bear in mind that the material presented here represents only single examples and is not representative. It was acquired in two case studies[5]: (1) an individual interview with the leader of a choir and (2) a group interview with volunteers doing pastoral counselling in a local parish (with supervision).

4 "[C]oreligionists may help define the problem situation, suggest a specific plan of action, and offer feedback and guidance as the plan is being executed." Neil M. Krause and Keith M. Wulff, "Friendship Ties in the Church and Depressive Symptoms: Exploring Variations by Age," *Review of Religious Research* 46 (2005): 325–340, 326.

5 Transcripts of the interviews are kept at the University of Tübingen, Germany. The following citations can be reviewed for scientific purposes.

2 "This upward openness, this is just really important to me": The Church Choir as an Offer for Participation

Ms. A (48 years old) has been the volunteer director of a church choir in a rural parish for 10 years; she spends about 8 hours per week on this task. Experiences within her family have raised her awareness of depression. Already at the beginning of the interview, she highlights that the members of the choir treat each other with care. "Everybody can be the way he or she is." This group atmosphere finds expression in them visiting each other in times of need. "Especially the women, certain women over and over again, they just take care of them, they just stop by there, they call them, and they ask what's going on." The choir leader sees herself in the role of a supporter she adapts the musical repertoire to the present group situation, asks for understanding for some and encourages others to come even when they are not feeling well. "I've already talked about the woman who broke into tears yesterday [. . .] it's really hard for her right now. She started to cry when we sang 'Lobe den Herrn' [a hymn of praise, 'Praise to the Lord'] too much, for example [. . .] and yesterday morning I met her, and I told her, you are allowed to cry, and then, the practice was over around 9:30 p.m., and 'til 11:00 I stood with her in front of the parish hall and talked to her."

The choir is not aiming for achievements but for participation and inclusion. "That's my goal, everybody should be allowed to sing with us. Even those should sing with us who cannot hold a note, or those who cannot read a note, and I always start with the basics, over and over again." Thus, what is important to her is "that feeling that I am welcome here, no matter how I'm feeling."

She understands this goal of her work to be an expression of her faith. On the one hand, this openness to everybody, also to "people who otherwise never go to church" is important to her, on the other hand also "this upward openness," which is reflected in the openness to everybody as well as in mutual responsibility as an integral part of her work. "I just feel responsible for my individual choir members. And I try to share this feeling, so all of them can carry a piece of responsibility with them."

This interview clearly shows that a choir is an easily accessible offering, which provides the possibility of experiencing community. But we can certainly not generalize this example. We can neither imply the same for other choirs in other congregations, nor can we deny groups outside of congregations the integrative effects that are highlighted here. It has, however, become apparent that the volunteer choir leader theologically reflects upon and interprets the social dimension of her choir. God's embracing of His people is supposed to be reflected in the way the choir members treat each other. "That feeling that I am welcome here, no matter how I'm feeling." This is how the choir leader understands her work, and she aligns this consciously with her principle: "Making belief tangible, that is the principle, of course."

Concerning depression, the emotionality that comes with the music is an important factor. The choir leader explains that besides of singing together, personal conversations about problems evolve: "music just softens one a bit." The collective singing creates a community, which "certainly feels good", even if it evokes tears. The community, which is "just" accompanied by "a joyful atmosphere" is always in the foreground.

The choir is essentially shaped by its leader's personality. During the interview, Ms. A freely talks about the importance of the support her minister shows for her work. One way this support is shown is by the clear approval of her ideas . . . "The best possible support I could have. So when I – when my brain – when I spin some idea again >laughs<; then, I can always go to my minister, and he will say 'yes, yes, yes, sounds good'!" She also generally feels that the focus on theology and church music together are also met with approval. She often mentions her minister's approval and how she feels "absolutely carried" by that. The parish council, on the other hand, does not always support her. "I'm a little worried about some in the parish council. They don't support me. That's very obvious and I wish they wouldn't block me, but that is new now. There are new people now in the parish council, and there is one person especially who blocks me a little, but, oh well."

The nature of the conflict is not explained in the interview, but Ms. A does not give much weight to it. The minister's support outweighs the lack of support from the parish council. The minister's position evokes the feeling of being "absolutely carried."

Of course, this interview represents not more than an individual perspective on the phenomenon of depression in a parochial context. Our research so far is only of a limited range, and we are at the very beginning of our evaluation. However, through careful evaluation of this interview, we can say that congregations can offer social support. Furthermore, social and religious functions are closely related. Choir leader A interprets her work explicitly in religious terms: the choir is a place where inclusion can be experienced, and so can the unconditional acceptance by God.

3 The Self-Conception of Volunteers Working in Pastoral Counselling: The Evaluation of a Group Interview

In the following a guided interview with a group of volunteers in a local congregation is eveluated. The group of five people already existed and had been meeting regularly for several years before our study began. Participants of the group are volunteer pastoral counselors in their congregation. Their group meetings serve as a platform for supervision and guidance. As part of the project "Kirchengemeinde und Depression" (Church Congregations and Depression),[6] they exchange information, plan events and invite guest speakers.

As opposed to individual interviews, group interviews offer the opportunity to reconstruct group communication and its patterns. This is especially significant for existing groups that are not created for a specific interview situation but already have a communicative practice and group culture shaped by shared routines and common experiences.[7] Because these group meetings serve also as 'counselling for counselors', group communication can be evaluated in terms of its therapeutic qualities. This is also the case during special circumstances, that is, when the group meeting is structured by interview questions and recorded.[8] The analysis of the interview follows the topics that structured the interview. The five participants were all female and the interview lasted for about 45 minutes.

3.1 "Yes, and then ... right, being at the right place": Pastoral Counselling as a Special Kind of Volunteer Work

The interviewees themselves connect the issue of motivation for volunteer work with what they are doing: spiritual care. While the interview guide was designed

---

6 Concerning this project with local congregation cf. chapter II.3. in this volume: Beate Jakob, *Is faith a Source of Strength? Do Congregations Offer Support? A Qualitative Study with People Affected by Mental Disorders and Their Relatives.*

7 Cf. the group interviews made in the context of the church membership study 4 (KMU 4) of the Protestant Church in Germany (EKD), cf. Jan Hermelink, Ingrid Lukatis and Monika Wohlrab-Sahr, *Kirche in der Vielfalt der Lebensbezüge. Die vierte EKD-Erhebung über Kirchenmitgliedschaft*, vol. 2, *Analysen zu Gruppendiskussionen und Erzählinterviews* (Gütersloh: Gütersloher Verlagshaus, 2006).

8 The guiding questions were developed by Beate Jakob, Annette Haußmann and Birgit Weyel. The interviews were conducted by Stefanie Zwanger and Annette Haußmann. The transcripts were made by Stephanie Zwanger and Johannes van Oorschot.

in a way that at first general motivation for volunteer work and then the specific motivation to volunteer in pastoral care should be discussed, participants reflected on their own motivation in the context of pastoral care. A1 opens the discussion: "My motivation is that I had a crisis some years ago . . . and I myself accepted some pastoral counselling and it was really good for me. And then, I decided if I should ever have the opportunity to do something like that, then I will do it. This ... was the reason ... for me." A3 immediately continues: "Yes, I think it's the same. For me it was pretty much the same . . . . So, I was a bit in a crisis and it helped me, and then I thought that I want to do the same, yes. If I can help others then . . . in this way, I like to do it, too." The positive experience with pastoral counselling during a personal crisis constitutes for A1 the reason to start volunteering ("and then, I decided . . . ") as it also does for A3. Both interviewees also connect the positive, personal experience with pastoral counselling with a self-assessment of being especially gifted as pastoral counselors themselves. Another interviewee also supports this motive. However, this claim to be especially gifted is not unproblematic – especially in a Christian context – because it can be (mis) understood as being bold and pretentious. The interviewer specifically asks A3 about a conversation outside of the interview: A3 apparently had claimed to have a special 'gift' for pastoral counselling. "Yes, you already said that in that line of work ... that you have a special gift there." A3 then chooses a much weaker phrasing. She places this insight in the context of her volunteer training and does not talk about the concept of being 'gifted' that has a religious connotation. "So, I was just sitting there during the training and thought, this is my thing." When more people during the interview agree and laugh, A3 phrases her thoughts more bluntly: "And then, simply, I know ah that I am ... yes, people often told me that I am good at pastoral counselling."

The interviewer then guides the conversation to the topic of the volunteer training. A1 confirms that all volunteers have to participate in this training before starting their volunteer work. After this clarification, A3 again picks up the previous topic and gives a biographical reason for her strong statement about her giftedness: "Well, yes, I actually have always been the one to talk to for her friends." When she moved to H. and was between jobs, she read the announcement for the preparation class for pastoral counselor volunteers. "Yes, I was part of it right from the beginning, quite enthusiastically ... yes, and then – it felt right, I felt like I was at the right place."

Up to this point A1 and A3 dominated the conversation, but now A5 speaks about the invitation to participate in the volunteer training. "For me it was the thing that . . . then the supervised spiritual counselling work was started. And I have done it more out of personal interest, for what was going to be there, and so on and so forth and that was really good, and ... ah ... and then it was the issue to continue the counselling and it happened that many things were done here in H., and I thought: okay, you should continue doing that – you like that. Yes, and then – then basically it was said that this is something I am good at (laughing)." By laughing, she cushions the statement about herself. Furthermore, A5 phrases the statement as did other people before her, which prevents the self-assessment to be seen as self-praise and in turn, open it up to be sanctioned. Pastoral counselling apparently requires specific credentials: three interviewees explicitly state a personal relationship to the subject matter and they stress more (A3) or less (A5) their competence in relation to experiences in their biography and perceptions of others about them ("it was said this is something I am good at"). All three stress how enthusiastically they pursue their volunteer work.

3.2 "And if you go to someone for pastoral counselling, you basically can say everything": On the Concept of Pastoral Care

What pastoral counselling is, highly depends on the people engaged in it. Content, roles and expectations are subject to negotiation among the participants. What people understand pastoral counselling to be, is embedded in concrete interactions and cannot be described definitively.[9] This is also true for professional pastoral care at counselling centers, in hospitals, or when pastors talk to people in the context of birthday visits, baptisms, funerals and such. In H., pastoral care done by volunteers is in principle not different from professional pastoral care. Volunteers have training in pastoral counselling, participate in supervision in group sessions on a regular basis and their work is officially recognized by the church. Thus, their work is different from other forms of day to day counselling that happens in the circle of friends and family.[10] However, it is also

9 Cf. Christoph Morgenthaler, *Seelsorge. Lehrbuch Praktische Theologie, Vol.* 3 (Gütersloh: Gütersloher Verlagshaus, 2009), 28: "Das, was Menschen jeweils unter Seelsorge und in diesem Zusammenhang unter Theologie, Gott und Religion verstehen, ist in gesellschaftliche Diskurse eingelagert, in welche diese Menschen eingebunden sind. Die Frage nach dem Wesen der Seelsorge kann auch definitorisch nicht einfach aufgelöst werden. Sie findet innerhalb unterschiedlicher Diskurse je wieder eine andere Antwort."

10 Wolfgang Steck makes clear that pastoral counselling is embedded in day to day communication and its structures, and professional pastoral counselling basically is a part of this culture of communication. "Es gibt viele Seelsorger auf der Bühne des Lebens. Der Pfarrer ist nur einer unter ihnen. Er übt die Seelsorge von Berufs wegen aus. Was den Pfarrer auszeichnet und ihn charakteristisch von den natürlichen Seelsorgern des Alltags unterscheidet, ist die besondere Kompetenz, die er sich durch seine Bildung und Ausbildung erworben hat. Die poimenische

not the same as professional counselling done by full- or part-time workers. Volunteer pastoral counselling has its own justification[11]– mostly carried by personal motives. Questions about the volunteers' self-conception are particularly interesting: How do they relate their work to professional pastoral counselling on the one hand, and day-to-day counselling among friends and family on the other hand? What are their particular strengths, and where are the limits of their work – especially concerning work with persons with mental disorders who have special requirements?

A5 responds to the interviewer's guiding question ("Why is pastoral care important to you?") by making a difference between pastoral care and other therapeutic services. She apparently thinks about psychological therapies when she says: "Because it is really problematic. So, there are many people having a crisis and it is a problem when they are looking for help. If they ... I don't know, want to start psychological therapy or something, there are long waiting periods." A waiting period can be bridged by pastoral counselling. "You can, you can at least if it's something difficult and somebody has to wait for his appointment with a psychologist, you can at least bridge the time." Here, pastoral counselling is not competing with psychological treatment or presents itself as an alternative to therapy but is bridging the gap until a professional therapy starts.

However, A5 also differentiates "if it is a quote unquote 'normal' life crisis, you know." This starts a conversation between A5 and A3 where they determine the differences between their own pastoral counselling and the day to day counselling with family members. A3 stresses that it is important "that someone can look at things neutrally. Because if you tell something to your own family, they might know all the people involved. And if it's some kind of relationship-story ... " A3 takes on the perspective of the affected people in describing the situation: "it's nice to have someone from the outside who doesn't know ... all the entanglements." A5 brings up another case where the opportunity to talk to friends or family does not exist. "But there simply are some people who have no one ... to talk to." But A3 points back to the systemic interdependencies that are important for counselling in everyday life. "Especially to talk openly, I think, . . . yes. Where you do not need to take precautions. Like, you know. Because this is your husband and so you cannot say everything. Or ... to your

Kompetenz ist allerdings wieder nichts anderes als eine spezifische Form des seelsorgerlichen Talents, über das jeder – in unterschiedlichem Maße freilich – verfügt." Wolfgang Steck, "Der Ursprung der Seelsorge in der Alltagswelt," *Theologische Zeitschrift 43* (1987): 175.

11 Cf. Jochen Schlenker, "Zur Sprache bringen," 273–288, especially 275f.

colleague you can't say everything. And if you go to someone in pastoral counselling, you can basically say everything."

In the context of these interviews, the concept of pastoral counselling is only connected to their own volunteer work. Both the professional therapeutic and medical services, and the 'talking and counselling' among friends, relatives, or colleagues are different. Pastoral counselling done by professionals, that is by ministers, is not mentioned at all. Volunteer pastoral counselling is counselling in the full sense of the word and does not need a further differentiation.

In the course of the discussion, the problem that people with mental disorders have to wait for long periods of time to begin a therapy is mentioned again. In this context, A1 brings up a new point: "[It's true] that there are many people who cannot afford a therapist. Very simple, yes. [...] And they are falling through the cracks and so there I see a mission for us as a congregation to be there for those people, right, who just cannot afford that but are in need, right. So often there is a dire need, right. And I think, we can actually do something there ... do something good and be there for those people."

3.3 "And simply to raise people's awareness": Talking about Depression as an Illness

The interviewer brings up depression as a topic because the group of volunteers has agreed to have an event[12] about it in their congregation. A4, who up to this point was not really engaged in the conversation, responds first, pointing to her personal involvement with the topic. "[S]o, it is a topic close to my heart because sadly I know it from my own family and I think that there is – you just start to listen differently or you just start to act differently with that." A2 adds that everyone can be hit by this illness: "I believe that everybody can get into such a situation, yes. If someone dies or you lose your job. So, nobody is immune to depression. Through circumstances of your live. You just lose the ground under your feet. And I think to help other people, or also ah ... to get out of there yourself by knowing more about it, that is also a great opportunity." A3 phrases it more generally: "So I think it is just a very common illness that despite this is still ... relatively hushed up." The issue of depression being a taboo is picked up by A1 who explains: "Well, I think especially within the

12 For information concerning the general project, see chapter II.3 in this volume: Beate Jakob, *Is Faith a Source of Strength? Do Congregations offer Support? A Qualitative Study with People Affected by Mental Disorders and their Relatives.*

congregation there is ah ... great shyness, too. I do not only recognize this in relation to depression, but more generally, ahh, to having a problem. Be it problems in relationships or ... what do I know ... So yes, people don't like to talk about difficult things or you have to ... yes, sometimes these are made into shameful topics. So this, I would say that. ... Yes. You have to be tough there." A1 reacts to the break in A3's sentence and continues: "you have to pray."

Taboo and shame, and to have a problem are connected to the Christian faith by this intervention and an interpretation for what A3 did not quite express is made. A3 then continues by saying: "So as Christians. Well as a Christian ... yes, life is supposed to be successful. So this, this tendency you can find again and again. Yes ... and then it is shameful if something goes wrong there, or depression is also this kind of, something nebulous, you don't know much about it, right, and it is scary, I think. There is ... I mean it starts with just a depressive mood." It becomes quite clear how well rehearsed this group is in their conversations. A1 reacts so sensitively that A3 can finish her thought. The topic of religion is put aside in the following argument. Instead, several interviewees talk extensively how difficult it was in some cases to make people understand that their problem is indeed an illness that needs treatment. A5 sums this up with precision: "Yeah. So, if I realize that I have a cold and then it turns into influenza then I go visit the doctor. And simply to raise people's awareness about that (i.e. depression), that is extremely important to me."

Consequently, the self-understanding of pastoral care in view of the issue "accepting the disease" is closely related to professional therapy. A1 tells the story, how difficult it was to convince a woman that she needed medical attention. "To accept the disease is the hardest thing. [humming] Yeah, that she eventually could really say: yes. I, I have a major depression, I need help, I will go to a hospital, that was hard work. Yes, I have to say that. She resisted for a long time."

3.4 "Sometimes you can only watch" – Pastoral Counselling and Experiencing Powerlessness

Following some extensive descriptions about the difficulties to understand depression as an illness that needs medical treatment, a new topic is brought up: the experience of being helpless. A4 talks about a woman, whose husband underwent medical treatment and whose doctor stopped the medication – at least according to the wife – relatively early. "And, ah, ... yes, I mean ... what can you say about that, yes, if the doctor says, okay, you don't need to take that medication anymore. Yes, of course you can go there and say, excuse me, don't you think it's a little early, yes. So I said to the women: I think it's a little early because it was a major depression." And indeed the illness worsened again. "Ah, you can ... that is the problem. You stand right next to it. You see where this is going, yes. And, ah ... sometimes you can only watch." A2 picks up that topic: "I think as well that depression is always connected to some kind of helplessness. Like, especially in families, or like that, there you experience, in my opinion, that ... that it spreads itself out. Well that, yes, that there is a great speechlessness [sound of a mobile phone] around that. I feel that this is really very ... very exhausting [muttering in the background] sometimes to endure that. This helplessness."[13]

Experiencing powerlessness is a central issue in the theory of pastoral care that is by no means limited to volunteers doing care work. The ambivalence of power and powerlessness in pastoral counselling also challenges professional counselors to deal with their own limitations and to reflect upon their professional and personal competences. Michael Klessmann reflects here on the role of counselors in hospitals who bring up topics of death and the limits of human life. "The position of a 'power-less-one' is not easy to bear: the role is unattractive, is not rewarded with attention or appreciation."[14] Reflecting upon one's own limits is an enormous challenge for each individual and stands in opposition to an important motive for volunteers doing pastoral care: the motive to help. "Volunteer workers want to do something meaningful and useful, to be needed and to shape the social live."[15]

3.5 "Praying does actually help," or: "he didn't want it in that moment": On the Ambivalence of Praying in the Context of Depression

The interviewer asks in what ways religious topics are relevant when counselling people with depression. A1 introduces prayer as a religious practice to the conversation: "Well, I for example, offer a prayer every time, ah, if people want

13 Cf. also the case study of Mrs. X in: Weyel, "Christian Communities in the Face of Immigration," 216–232, 223.

14 Michael Klessmann, "Macht und Ohnmacht in Seelsorge und Beratung," *WzM* 67 (2015): 344–357, 356f (trans. Birgit Weyel).

15 Jochen Schlenker, "Zur Sprache bringen," 273–288, 275. Cf. as well Stephan Seidelmann, *Evangelische engagiert – Tendenz steigend. Sonderauswertung des dritten Freiwilligensurveys für die Evangelische Kirche, Sozialwissenschaftliches Institut der EKD* (Hannover: EKD, 2012), 18 (trans. Birgit Weyel).

it. And up to now, no one has declined. Yes. Yes, it is interesting and as well, the feedback mostly is: this was really good for me now. Yes ... (clapping, audible exhale) ... How much, well, I don't believe that if somebody has a real depression only prayer would help – that's not what I want to say with this. (Laughing) But prayer does actually help. Now. Whatever the situation a person is in, if he wants to make use of it. So, I experience that it brings relief and helps, it is help." The interviewer then brings up possible negative aspects of religion, like a negative image of God as a God that only punishes. A4 tells the story of a women, for whom the issue of guilt was most pressing. A4 then, referring to A1, also brings up the possibility of praying. "Ah, when I am at the point where, where ... – I didn't have that case, but certainly you come to the point when you say, okay so ... I don't know how to continue here, I can only think of praying, then that is the case, yes. Well, then I would say the same, yes. But I think it is important ... to have respect when a person does not want praying." The interviewer again pushes the issue that with the illness of depression there is the possibility to feel you have lost your connection to God, "that a person who is depressed somehow has lost his or her faith." A2 responds to this position by insisting how dangerous this illness is because it often leads to suicide. She stresses again that "one [the volunteer] then goes with the person ... to a therapist, someone in practice or to pass this on to someone so that you don't start to interfere in the doctor's territory." She possibly thought that the question was meant critically and now tries to prevent the impression that the volunteers take the illness too lightly when they pray with and for the affected. A5 then again supports the point made by A4 that prayer is indeed a positive option even in the situation of pastoral counselling with a person suffering from depression. "But in the particular case, if someone loses his faith during his depression. I think then it can be ... helpful to say that there is this 'believing for someone' and that ah (2) that you actually pray for him, yes, that you stand in for him and ... and I actually think that this is helpful for those people, yes. If they can't find words ... that someone does it for them. I think that this is really ... very helpful."

A2 reacts more critically to the issue. Although a different opinion is expressed, all group members show great respect for one another. A2: "You have to know. So, I, at the moment, I know, I know someone who does not want that at the moment." A5 immediately adds: "yes ... of course." A2 continues to express the problem she feels: "So the, the, the, so what, if he is in a depression or not, but he suffers so much at the moment that he says: I don't want to have anything to do with that. I don't understand that and I don't want that either. And he would think of it as imposed upon him or something like that. So he, so I think you have to be so sensitive to say: ah ... ah, I am leaving this out.

Because if you recognize t- t- that he cannot work with that. Because he is so far away."

The interview sequence about prayer illustrates that it is indeed possible to have and to express controversial opinions connected to different styles of piety. This is only possible in a group that is based on mutual respect and trust and is supported by the group's participation in supervision. And indeed, this group has been together for many years. They know each other and have a routine in their exchanging of arguments. At various times, it has been pointed out that this kind of training-group is an important motivation for volunteers working in pastoral care.[16] "This motivation cannot be underestimated, because it can carry the demotivating experiences working in pastoral counselling and prevents that the people who are counselled are used for self-motivation."[17]

4 Conclusion

Both examples of volunteer pastoral care give clear insight into the self-conception of volunteer pastoral care workers in local congregations. An interesting finding is that, in the case of the choir leader, pastoral care is done "on the side". The "pastoral care", provided by communal singing in the congregation, is supported and accompanied by reflections of the choir leader: her attentiveness to the group and her reflected dealing with the effects of singing. Pastoral care is the implicit and at the same time, overriding goal of the choir work – explicitly reflected upon in the theological conception of her work ("this upward openness"). Following this example, it would be an interesting question whether other areas of volunteer work can also be identified in this way as pastoral care and thus get the attention they deserve. Eberhard Hauschildt pointed out that the work of volunteers – even if happening in settings like visiting groups that are similar to professional pastoral care – are not explicitly conceptualized as pastoral care[18] but rather as diaconal or missionary work. For a practical theology of volunteer-pastoral-care, we need to focus on the effects of pastoral

16 Regina Rhode, *Supervision und Ehrenamt – Welche Rahmenbedingungen, Fort- und Weiterbildung brauchen Ehrenamtliche für ihre Arbeit und was kann die Supervision dazu beitragen? Am Beispiel der Ehrenamtlichen Evangelischen Klinikseelsorge der Universitätsklinik Freiburg. Masterthesis, Evangelische Hochschule Freiburg, Masterstudiengang Supervision*, in URL: http://arhode.de/regina/files/Masterthesis_ReginaRhode.pdf (last accessed on 1 April 2020), 26.

17 Jochen Schlenker, "Zur Sprache bringen," 273–288, 277.

18 Cf. Eberhard Hauschildt, "Auf dem Weg zu einer Praktischen Theologie der Ehrenamtlichen-Seelsorge. Eine Skizze," *Pastoraltheologie* 99 (2010): 116–127, 122, fn. 25.

care in these lines of work without ignoring the other dimensions which have been mentioned.

The group interview on the other hand, gave insight into the self-conception of a group of volunteers working explicitly as "volunteer pastoral counselors". Their work is – apart from the structural conditions – not different from professional pastoral counselling. One could indeed say it is "semi-professional pastoral counselling"[19] that is not different in terms of its quality standards. The interview shows that the clarity of the role and the ability to reflect on experiences meets professional levels. The observation that limitations and boundaries of their work are defined in light of professional medical and psychiatric competences rather than those of ministers reflects the shared level of professionalism.

And indeed, the difference between the two is not that pastoral counselling itself is more or less limited but rather that the volunteer workers do not need to set the structural conditions of their work – but this is done by the professionals that choose volunteers and are responsible for the quality of their training. To honour all the work in the field of pastoral care in local congregations, it remains – following Eberhard Hauschild[20]– an important issue to also include all those who implicitly engage in pastoral counselling in everyday life, such as everyday social interactions, but nonetheless with caring effects.

19 Hauschildt, "Auf dem Weg zu einer Praktischen Theologie," 116–127, 125.
20 Hauschildt, "Auf dem Weg zu einer Praktischen Theologie," 116–127, 126.

Beate Jakob

Is Faith a Source of Strength? Do Congregations Offer Support?

A Qualitative Study with People Affected by Mental Disorders and their Relatives

1 Introduction

There is plenty of literature documenting that alongside a professional therapy, social support and spirituality can have a positive impact on the course of mental disorders.[1]

The Chair for Practical Theology with focus on Pastoral Care and Pastoral Theology at the Faculty of Protestant Theology, University of Tübingen, and the German Institute for Medical Mission (DIFÄM) designed a research project[2] to find out if individuals living with mental disorders and their relatives actually benefit from their personal faith and/or receive support from congregations. A qualitative study was performed using a semi-structured interview guide.

The research questions were:

- Do congregations support the interviewed people living with mental disorders and their relatives?
- Is personal faith a source of strength for the interviewed people living with mental disorders and their relatives?
- Do the interviewees have a religious interpretation of their disease vs. the disease of their relatives?

The interviewees were found by purposive sampling. Eleven persons volunteered to answer the questions. Among them were five persons living with a mental disorder (A 1–5; 3 women, 2 men) and six relatives (B 1–6; 5 women, 1 man).

With the consent of the interviewees, the interviews were recorded and transcribed. The evaluation was done by content analysis.

1 See the chapters in the first part of this volume (I. Religion and Health – An Overview).

2 The research was part of the project "Congregations and Mental Health" which was conducted by the Department for Practical Theology III of the Faculty of Protestant Theology, University Tübingen, and the German Institute for Medical Mission (DIFÄM) in cooperation with health professionals forming an "Alliance against Depression" ("Bündnis gegen Depression").

https://doi.org/10.1515/9783110674217-007

The methodology of narrative interviews was chosen because we wanted to learn more about the experiences of those who are directly affected by mental disorders. The questions initiated the narration and allowed for a wide range of experiences. But they also focused the contents on the main research questions of our project: the impact of congregations and the assessment of faith and the interplay between faith and dealing with the disease. Most of the interviewees have been living with mental disorders for a long time. They went through many phases and experienced ups and downs which activated coping strategies. In some respects, the interviewees disclose expert knowledge regarding people affected and their relatives.

The interviewer[3] adopted an attitude of appraisal and empathy. The texts of the transcripts were broken down by the methodology of reconstructive social research, basically encoding according the qualitative content analysis with an emphasis on in-vivo-codes.[4]

2 Interviews with People Living with Mental Disorders

All interview partners mention their diagnosis during the interview: Four are living with depression, one with a schizoaffective disorder (A 2). In a first part of the interviews, the respondents shared how their disease affects their daily lives and their relationship with others.

2.1 Living with a Mental Disorder

2.1.1 "Just nothing"

All interview partners have been sick for a long time and the disorders have a significant impact on their lives. Three of them mentioned frequent suicidal thoughts in the past.

---

3 Stefanie Koch conducted the interviews. She also prepared the transcripts and published a summary of the content. Cf. in: Beate Jakob and Birgit Weyel, eds., *Menschen mit Depression. Orientierungen und Impulse für die Praxis in Kirchengemeinden* (Gütersloh: Gütersloher Verlagshaus, 2014), 54–67.

4 Cf. Udo Kuckartz, *Qualitative Inhaltsanalyse. Methoden, Praxis, Computerunterstützung* (Weinheim and Basel: Beltz Juventa, ^{2}2014); Udo Kuckartz, *Einführung in die computergestützte Analyse qualitativer Daten* (Wiesbaden: VS Verlag für Sozialwissenschaften, ^{3}2010).

At the time of the interview, none of the interviewees was employed. Asked about the main symptoms of the disorder during an acute phase, A 1 says: "Just lying in bed. No drive at all [...] there were times when I was rarely able to wash a salad [...] no joy, no emotions; and the worst is when there is just emptiness, nothing, even no negative feelings, just nothing." She reports about two suicidal attempts.

A 5 feels empty and weak during an acute phase of depression. "The biggest decision to make is getting up in the morning," says A 4.

A 3 talks about his feelings and behavior during phases of depression: "Loneliness and withdrawal [...] fasting." He avoids any social contact by building up a "wall" around himself as he does not want anybody to know about his condition.

2.1.2 Lack of Understanding and Social Isolation

Still today, mental disorders are often not regarded as diseases but as conditions that can be controlled by one's will power. Lack of knowledge about mental disorders is still widespread in our society. The interview partners know about this deficit: "People who are not affected [by mental disorders] don't have any idea about depression and other mental illnesses" (A 3).

People living with mental disorders feel misunderstood by others, even by their relatives. According to A 1, most people cannot understand that persons younger than themselves fall mentally ill. When staff of the local 'Diakoniestation' came to assist her, a neighbour asked, "Do they wash you?" At that time, she was 30 years old. Furthermore, even after 22 years of her illness, her own mother has not understood the nature of depression, and her husband has not been helpful to her. Even family members expect them to pull themselves together, to just do something instead of being weak, etc. It is also not helpful to hear phrases like, "Cheer up", "It's going to get better [...]" (A 4).

Therefore, the interviewees wish information to be provided about mental disorders and their disease character. People should understand that "though not having a physical impairment, a person with depression is not able to get up in the morning and, for example, is not able to brush his or her teeth" (A 3).

Lack of knowledge resulting in misunderstanding sometimes leads to exclusion and even stigmatization of people living with mental disorders. It is a painful experience, "If you realize that people turn away; if you realize that they talk about you or judge you because you are not able to act" (A 1). She also mentions that somebody said, "Obviously, one actually cannot talk with mentally sick persons." A 5: "It hit me when some friends turned away from me; all of a sudden, they didn't want anything to do with me anymore." She even regards social isolation as a factor causing or sustaining her mental disorder: "Being here so isolated [...] I am sure this is one of the reasons why I have this [the mental disorder]."

2.1.3 What Helps?

All interview partners are in professional treatment, and they all see the need for treatment. But A 4 sees that drugs were not a magic bullet for him. In the same line, all respondents acknowledge other factors have also had an impact on the course of their disease. It is, e.g., very important that there is a good disease management which should be coordinated by a psychiatrist (A 1).

The significance of social factors is mentioned frequently. A 4 says: "Medication is not a magic bullet that can cure mental disorders if we only rely on it, but has to be complemented, particularly through social contacts offering the possibility to talk."

During phases of severe depression, the interview partners tend to withdraw and to be on their own. At the same time, they know that – particularly after periods of being severely sick – talking to and being in community with others is necessary and has a healing potential. "Talking, talking, talking [...] about oneself, about other issues [...] to try to be in contact with others" (A 1) is helpful.

During serious phases of illness, the affected persons are not able to expose themselves to others. This should be understood, even by friends, says A 2. Still, a phone call might be appreciated as this shows her that she has not been forgotten. However, the caller should not start the conversation by asking 'How are you', because (A 2), "What can I answer to this question when I feel bad?" Instead, one could start by saying, e.g., "I'd just like to get in touch with you."

Three persons very much value being members of a self-help group. This is because there is a basic even non-verbal understanding among the members of these groups. Moreover, one hears from others how they are, "You can share, and one gets tips" (A 1). They also highlight positively that from time to time speakers are invited to talk about topics related to mental health (A 5). For A 2, the main benefit of the group is getting in touch with others.

2.2 Is the Local Congregation a Place where You Find Support? Does Your Faith Help You?

As a social network in general the congregation is appreciated, but the question arises if it is a place where people with mental disorders feel supported.

2.2.1 Spiritual and Social Support

A 1 is member of a local congregation and benefits from it. Since she fell sick, she has received help from some pastors. During the first phase, a pastor of a neighbouring congregation counselled her and her husband. The pastor of the congregation she now belongs to has repeatedly assisted her, e.g. by advising her when she searched for another psychotherapist, or by organizing practical help for her household while she was in the hospital. Moreover, he regularly organizes events and invites speakers to sensitize and inform the congregation members about mental health and mental disorders.

In her congregation, she is a member of a women's group. She takes part in the meetings even when she is very ill. Though not being able to listen properly to a talk that is given, she nevertheless is integrated in the group.

She likes to attend the Sunday service as it strengthens her and also because she meets friends there. At the time of the interview, however, she cannot make it: "I am trying to get up, but then go to bed again. This is a pity as it has always brought me a lot." Therefore, she would be happy about offers taking place later during the day. A meditation group that used to meet in the evening does not exist anymore.

During the first years of her illness, she had strong feelings of guilt, and these feelings led to frequent suicidal thoughts. But over time, she learnt how to avoid such an interpretation of her illness. Today, she strictly denies having any religious interpretation of it. Her faith helps her to cope with her illness: "All in all, faith helps me. But there were times when I was not able to pray at all, so that I could not even say the Lord's Prayer. After two sentences I was distracted and trapped in my brooding. But, in the [name] hospital in 1995, I had such an experience after I had been totally down for days and everything had been so empty and bad. I walked into the forest and then there was a ray of sunshine and then I had such a feeling and thought this to be a sign from above and [...] only very briefly, but this was very beautiful."

As she cannot manage to attend the Sunday service, she prays and reads the Moravian Daily Texts and tries to say the Lord's Prayer.

2.2.2 "This ruined my life"

One of the interview partners (A 4) had a very traumatizing experience with his local congregation, particularly with the pastor. It still upsets him: When he was young, his mother suffered from a psychosis and sometimes disturbed the Sunday mass through her strange behavior. In his preaching, the pastor called mental disorders a punishment from God. The pastor's statements from the pulpit hit him very hard and put a lot of pressure on him so that he even doubted if he actually had a right to exist. "This ruined my life [...] saying that this is a punishment of God or something like this, is almost a death sentence. [...] It just hit me very much. And still I have difficulties with it, maybe in my subconscious mind," he says. He goes so far as to say that "This guy [the pastor] still upsets me [...] he should have been taken to court." It is his hope that pastors today think differently about mental disorders.

Nevertheless, he clearly differentiates between the church and religion: "I would not ban religion [...] as I then would deprive people of something that eventually can help them a bit." Visiting towns or villages for the first time, he usually goes to the church. There he sits quietly and meditates. Though his earlier experiences still affect him, he himself denies any religious interpretation of his illness.

2.2.3 Material Benefits

A 3 has benefitted from his congregation as his electricity bill was paid by them when he could not cover it. As he considers the church to be very rich, he challenges the church to practice its diaconal mandate by supporting people with mental disorders financially and also by offering them jobs. Beyond expecting practical help from the church, he does not seem to take the spiritual dimension into account.

Another respondent (A 5), would also appreciate the churches to provide little tasks for people with mental disorders and should pay them something. Besides the money that might help the people, she thinks this is a matter of appreciation and restoring people's dignity.

2.2.4 Experiences in a Free Church

A 2 was a member of a mainline church. There, she feels that "one doesn't disclose but wants to keep a mental disorder to oneself." Since some time, she has been attending a free church. The vibrancy of the services and the modern songs attract her. She prays every morning and evening, and she says: "Yes – this [my faith] keeps me together." She is sure she would be worse off without her faith. While she herself has no religious interpretation of her illness, the free church she is in contact with does. They regard illnesses not being from God but from evil. She also shared about her difficult experiences with another lady at the free church. After it became known that she was affected by a mental disorder, she was treated badly and was no longer allowed to continue with her task in the congregation – she had been working with children.

2.2.5 Longing for Social Support

While not being an active member of a congregation, A 5 longs to being included in a church community. She says: "I almost envy a friend who tells me that on Sundays, in her church, they have coffee together, they, the congregation members, sit together. She is firmly included in the congregation. Such a community is what I miss! I don't have it. [...] I long for a community where I am part of, but such a community is not there in [name of her congregation] [...] A group should be formed; it should meet continuously instead of only once or twice a year. Such a group should just be initiated."

3 Does the Congregation Support You? Does Your Faith Help You? Voices of Relatives

All relatives who volunteered to be interviewed are very much involved with their relatives' mental disorders. Two of them live with a schizoaffective disorder, and four with depression. They all mention past or present feelings of helplessness and that it is extremely stressful to accompany sick children or to live with a person who suffers without being able to change their condition. Is faith a help for the interviewees and are they supported by a congregation? And do they have a religious interpretation of their relatives' disease?

3.1 "Sometimes I can no longer believe."

B 1 has a son who has been suffering from a psychosis for ten years. For him as well as for his wife it has been very hard to endure the suffering of their son without being able to help him. As a young man, he himself had had phases of psychosis. For the past ten years, their life has been dominated by their son's illness. Only now, as he has improved a bit, they can think about other things and live their own life.

B 1 is a retired pastor. He has thought a lot about how to integrate his son's illness in his relationship with God. This has been a struggle up to today:

"Sometimes, I can no longer believe." There were also times when he felt guilty of his son's illness, asking himself what he missed during his son's childhood. These feelings were so strong and put him under such pressure that he himself visited a psychotherapist and took antidepressants. The sessions with the therapist as well as the medication helped him a lot.

There were also phases when he was angry with God and even hated him and was outraged about his situation. Martin Luther's statement 'the sons who hate and blaspheme him during temptations, God loves most' has helped him. But still, his faith is often tested and he cannot understand the discrepancy between reality and the 'Good News' of the New Testament. He is of the opinion that the promise "Whoever believes in him may have eternal life" (John 3: 15)[5] includes the promise of being healed including physical health.

He knows that "one never can understand God and his plans", and he is convinced that still it is the best for him to stay with God: "It is better to believe than not to believe. [...] As there is no other option, I stay with him."

Though he is retired, he still likes to hold services in congregations from time to time. Whenever he prepares a sermon, he actually addresses himself. For example, it helped him to meditate on the biblical story of Joseph and his brothers that ends with the statement: "You meant evil against me; but God meant it for good" (1 Moses 50:20).[6] To him, the story tells a kind of basic trust in God and his good will – "This is what I would like to develop further." He agrees to biblical verses like: "It is good that one should wait quietly for the salvation of the Lord" (Lamentations 3:26).[7]

Based on his personal experience, the interviewee advocates for a strong focus on pastoral theology in theological education: "I think that [...] with regard to theology, pastoral counselling has to be re-evaluated [...] The pastor has to be the local doctor for the soul." According to him, only a sermon including pastoral aspects can actually help people.

3.2 "Miracles still happen"

For 19 years, B2 has been accompanying her husband who lives with a schizoaffective disorder. For her, it has been difficult to bear with her own helplessness. Sometimes, it was like her husband lived behind a wall so that she could not

5 The Holy Bible: English Standard Version (ESV).
6 The Holy Bible: (ESV).
7 The Holy Bible: (ESV).

reach him. She also mentions that she had difficulties accepting the illness as it started so suddenly: "It was like the whole thing [...] hit us, and I had no idea how it was going to develop, and definitely I had no idea that this [his condition] was a mental disorder. I didn't agree with him that he should take an antidepressant. And I talked him out of that." During periods when he was severely sick, she had to teach him to manage the simplest activities like washing and shaving himself.

In retrospect, she thinks she was not properly informed and supported by the doctors and therapists. She felt they did not want her to interfere with their therapy. The support groups for relatives helped her while other people, even her friends, were not supportive. It affected her very negatively when a friend said: "It would have been better if he [her husband] had died."

Unlike her husband, B 2 was brought up as a Christian. Both of them do not have any affiliation to a congregation now. Asking for help from congregation members, therefore, has never been an option for her.

Though not having any affiliation with a congregation, she notes that "Let me say that nobody from the congregation came to me [...] Nobody even tried." This is also true for a neighbour, who is very much involved in her congregation and with whom she had a good relationship. But she also admits that if the neighbour had sent somebody from the church to them, her husband certainly would have said: "Thanks for your offer, but I don't want you to come." During his stays in the hospital they met two chaplains, but they did not like either of them.

Faith is not a source of strength for her but she admits that it is different for others. She knows a woman whose daughter suffered from a mental disease and died. The woman is faithful and an active member of a congregation. She sings in the church choir. This woman often mentions that her only comfort is to know her daughter is with God where she now is in good hands.

B 2 denies any religious interpretation of her husband's illness as she is "a rational person". However, without giving an explicit religious interpretation, she had kind of religious thoughts when her husband got better after a long period of illness: "When I saw him taking a newspaper and reading it for the first time after years, I thought that 'Miracles still happen'. We are both not Christians, but somehow I thought that this came somehow from heaven." She connoted this statement with a laugh.

3.3 In the congregation, "you know too many people"

B 3 shares that six years ago her son disclosed that he suffered from depression and had to take medication. Although he asked her to keep it secret, she told all her relatives about his disorder. She as well as her son were very much supported by their family, and she also appreciates being a member of the support group for relatives. Initially, she blamed herself for not having noticed her son becoming sick and said to herself: "What kind of mother you are as you haven't realized your child is sick!" Moreover, she was very insecure of how to behave and interact with him. In this regard, the family and the support group helped her a great deal.

During almost all of her professional life, B 3 taught religious education. She goes to church on a regular basis but she is not a member of church groups like dancing groups for elderly people and the like. Her local congregation does not provide any offers for people with mental disorders. B 3 affirms that her personal faith is highly important for her. For her, it is a source of strength and helps her to cope with the situation. But she would not address the pastor or anybody else in the congregation to talk about her problems. In this regard, she refers to a friend whose daughter has a mental disease. This friend would never disclose in her congregation as "You know too many people there and you don't want to pillory this [the disease]."

B 3 strictly denies any religious interpretation of mental disorders. She regards them as metabolic diseases comparable to physical diseases: "If you break your leg, you also don't say that this is God's will or something like this."

3.4 Spiritual Support Outside the Church

For 40 years, the husband of B 4 has been living with depression accompanied by frequent suicidal thoughts. For years, B 4 had always been afraid of finding her husband dead. In the meantime, she learnt that she cannot hinder him from committing suicide if he definitely wants to do so.

Her husband is very shy and fearful, and he avoids social contacts. He even rarely talks to his own children. Life in itself seems to be a burden to him and he cannot act spontaneously. It is her task to plan their life and she takes all responsibility while she sometimes longs for a husband she could rely on. Asked how she can cope with the condition of her husband, she says: "At times well, at times badly." Nobody helped her except one doctor. While her husband was being treated by him, the doctor also cared for her and she felt he understood her. Other people including their relatives showed little understanding. They said things to him like, "Hey, pull yourself together."

B 4 still well remembers difficult childhood experiences. When she was preparing to celebrate her First Holy Communion, the parish priest told her that her parents would not be allowed to receive the Holy Communion as they had remarried after divorce. As she loved her parents very much she absolutely could not understand such a statement and was very upset. Since that time she has lost her confidence in the church. Accordingly, the congregation is not a place for her to go to. However, she and her husband had very helpful conversations with a lay theologian ("Pastoralreferent") working in a parish. He visited them and told them that mental disorders are medical conditions. He helped them to overcome feelings of guilt. To her, this shows that it depends on the particular person you talk to if it is helpful or not. She adds, "I think it is most important that somebody offers his time and gives you the feeling he is happy to do so. Because you just feel if this is the case."

Her faith helps B 4 very much to cope with the situation: "Very much indeed. I have my guardian angels [. . .] and the Lord's Prayer, particularly the 'Your will be done', is very important to me [. . .] It is every day that I think that 'if Your will is done then it is the right will', and then it goes just on, yes."

Nature is also a source of strength for her: "Let me say I am not a church goer. I definitely can't go to church; this doesn't bring me anything. But if I go out for a walk in the morning which I usually do almost every day, if I go out into the nature and everything is so beautiful, this is like 100 churches for me. [. . .] this is so good. Or going to swim early in the morning, then there is an atmosphere that you just think to be in paradise, yes." In addition, her hobby of stone carving is a kind of spiritual experience as it is like meditating on her own life.

She denies a religious interpretation of her husband's illness. However, it bears a meaning for herself: "I keep thinking that it is my task to accompany him [her husband] and to walk with him as long as possible." During the decades of his illness, there were periods when she was desperate and at the same time very angry with her husband. Sometimes she nearly felt like she wanted to beat him. She was deeply ashamed of these feelings and shared them with a spiritual counselor. The counselor told her that she was allowed to be angry, as her anger was a kind of protection for her. She was very relieved as he told her: "Don't be angry with yourself, because you need it."

3.5 Potentials of Congregations

The daughter of B 5 was 19 years old when she fell into depression for the first time. That was 13 years ago. For the past eight years she has stayed off medication. However, her condition is not stable; often, she is stressed and overworked, and then she complains about headaches and muscle tensions. For a couple of years, B 5 felt very isolated and lonely. Even with her husband she could not always share her feelings as he was not willing to put the illness of their daughter at the centre of his life as she did. He regarded the illness under a medical and more rational aspect while she was deeply emotionally affected. She then found help in the relatives' support group. There she could, e.g. share a letter from her daughter in which she blamed the parents for her illness. The group members could calm her down by saying that it was understandable that young people seek an explanation for their illness.

Religion and faith do not help her, says B 5. She denies any religious interpretation of her daughter's illness. However, she says: "Faith would have helped me, if I had had it. [...] I very much envied all those in the group [support group for relatives] who had such a strong faith because they were held while I was like swimming."

B 5 is not member of a congregation and does not seek help from there. But she clearly sees a big potential of how congregations could help people with mental disorders and their relatives. Based on talks with relatives, she knows that they are looking for a place to go to, and they ask themselves if a congregation might be such a place. Many would appreciate a conversation with the pastor. Moreover, relatives are in need of relaxation exercises or meditation: "This would have helped us during periods when we felt so bad." Just meditating in an adult evening class is not the same; she would have prefered a meditation grounded in spirituality.

She also mentions that people living with mental disorders wish to be integrated in the congregation: "Some kind of work they can be involved or just be of help anywhere in the congregation, e.g. as members of the choir or if they help to serve coffee during meetings in the afternoon or something like that. [...] But the initiative should come from the parish as they themselves are without drive."

3.6 The Congregation "is not integrated in my life"

B 6 did not want to accept the fact when her husband developed a depression 1 ½ years ago: "I defended myself against it [the disease], because I didn't want to believe it." The illness is still like a taboo within her family. Instead of asking her husband how he is, the relatives turn to her if they want to know about him. She thinks they are afraid to say something wrong. When she attended a support group, she felt burdened instead of finding relief because the members shared very frightening experiences with relatives suffering from severe psychoses. The only person she had helpful conversations with was the leader of the support group.

Asked about faith, B 6 explains, "Well, I do believe in something but I would not say that I am faithful in the ecclesiastical sense [. . .] But I believe that everything in life has somehow a meaning . . . that nothing happens without any reason [. . .] and that if you have to endure such things, that this then again does something positive. [. . .] and can become something beautiful. This is what I can hold on to." She refuses any religious interpretation of her husband's illness: "I don't believe that this is a kind of fate or given by God or so – no, this I don't believe."

For her, the congregation is not a place to go to: "I don't have any connection to the congregation. Actually, it is not integrated in my life. Therefore, it would have never come to my mind to contact the congregation." She does not deny that congregations can provide helpful offers for relatives of people with mental disorders. However, she thinks she herself would not use them.

4 Summary and Conclusion

People living with mental disorders and relatives often feel they are misunderstood by others and isolated as there is still a widespread lack of sound knowledge about the characteristics of mental disorders.

None of the five interviewees living with mental disorders denied the importance of professional treatment. At the same time, however, all pointed to the positive impact of social support. In line with this, one person believes that social isolation to be a causative factor for her illness. For three of them a self-help group provides a social network. Only one interviewee feels supported by her congregation. For the others, the congregation is not a place they expect or actually receive support. One respondent mentions an example of a congregation that has a focus on social interaction and she would very much appreciate being part of such a community. In addition to being a social network, the congregations might offer people with mental disorders little paid jobs that help them to regain self-confidence.

The same is true for relatives of people living with mental disorders. They do not receive support from congregations. However, one of them who is not a member of a congregation sees lots of possibilities for congregations to be of relevance for people living with mental disorders as well as for the relatives, e.g. by offering meditation groups. Two interview partners living with a mental disorder pray on a regular basis. They perceive their personal faith as a source of strength. A man who had very difficult experiences with a pastor, still sees that one has to differentiate between church and personal faith. He does not deny that faith can help and shares about his practice of visiting churches and meditating there.

One of the relatives is a theologian who struggled with God and went a long way to integrate his son's disease with his faith. All the relatives are willing to talk about faith issues and see faith as a possible source of strength. One says that faith keeps her together while another admits that faith would have helped her if she had had it. None of them is of the opinion that faith might cause mental disorders or can have a negative impact on them.

Presently, none of the respondents has a religious interpretation of his or her disease or the disease of their relatives. One mentions feelings of having been guilty in the past which she has totally overcome. Even a man who when he was young was exposed to a pastor preaching about the connection between mental disorders and personal guilt has completely freed himself from this opinion.

In conclusion, the interviews showed that personal faith can complement a professional therapy. While the majority of the interviewees do not receive support from a congregation, there is a large potential in this regard. The classical way of offering pastoral counselling is still very important. Hosting self-help groups and support groups for relatives are other possibilities. However, a congregation should also think about offers people can take part in without disclosing their personal needs. Of course, every Sunday service is an invitation for people who are not well off. But, in addition, meditation groups, Bible groups, open women groups, singing and dancing groups might be attractive for people with mental disorders. These groups combine spirituality and social support without exclusively addressing people in need.

In addition to offering social and spiritual support, congregations can address the knowledge gap about mental disorders that prevails in our society. Thematic Sunday services, lectures about mental health, and inviting people living with mental disorders to openly talk about their disease are just a few means to sensitize about mental health issues and provide sound information about the disease character of mental disorders.

Annette Haußmann, Beate Jakob, and Birgit Weyel

Spirituality, Congregational Support, and Mental Health: The Example of Depression

Results of a Comparative Study among Volunteers in Congregations and Professionals in Health Care Settings, Conducted in Germany and Malawi

1 Introduction

In line with the concept of congregations owning health assets and based on the assumption that spirituality can have a positive effect on health, the following study was conducted in Germany and Malawi to present a comparison. Once again, depression was taken as an example as it is one of the most common mental disorders worldwide and because there is a treatment gap between the countries of the Global North and in the Global South. Congregations, so the basic assumption, can be an important resource for those who do not know much about depression as well as for those who are looking for help for their mental problems. Confronted with mental disorders, pastors and voluntary workers in pastoral care without any training in mental health often do not know how to deal with these problems.

In this study, we tried to link research about voluntary work from a motivational perspective with attitudes concerning the relationship between health and religiosity. We were interested to learn about any differences in the perception of this relationship as exist in Malawi and Germany, which are countries with quite different health care systems and cultures. The comparison is of interest because the approach of assets related to congregations and volunteers provides a connecting factor. Nevertheless, one must keep in mind that a comparison between quite different cultures and situations is very limited.

https://doi.org/10.1515/9783110674217-008

2 The Study in Germany

2.1 Aim and Research Questions

The project focuses on the motives of volunteers in pastoral care, their mind-set and attitudes toward the relationship between mental health and religiosity, and the role of a church congregation. Accordingly, the study addressed three different aspects:

1. Why do people engage in voluntary work concerning pastoral care in a congregation? What is their personal motivation to be involved in a project on depression?
2. What are their attitudes towards the impact of religiosity and church congregations on people living with depression?
3. How do they interpret the relationship between church congregation and health (religious meaning concepts)?

2.2 Methods and Results

Methods: A questionnaire comprised of three different parts according to the main questions of the study was applied. In the first part, questions about the individual motivation to volunteer were asked. The second part contained questions about the role of the congregation regarding support for mental health problems in general. Personal faith opinions and religiosity were assessed with the scale of centrality (Z-Scale[1]). Characteristics of the participants (age, gender, role in the congregation, experience with depression) followed at the end of the questionnaire.

Participants: 59 volunteers from 3 different congregations participated. They all attended a training course in their congregation to learn more about depression, its symptoms, possibilities of therapy and conversation techniques. Most of them were already engaged in some kind of pastoral care group. At the end of this course, they were asked to complete a questionnaire. The characteristics are shown in Table 1.

1 Stefan Huber and Odilo W. Huber, "The Centrality of Religiosity Scale (CRS)," *Religions* 3 (2012): 710–724.

Table 1: Characteristics of the German sample.

Characteristics	**Results in Germany (percent)**
Role in the church congregation	46 Volunteers with different professional backgrounds participating in group training (78%) 5 members of local pastoral care teams (8%) 8 members of the local project team organizing depression related events (14%)
Gender	81% female, 19% male
Age	M = 54.6 years (SD = 11.04 years, min 34, max 78)
Church affiliation	34% very much associated 46% rather associated 18% somehow associated 2% barely associated
Religiosity (scale of centrality, Z-Scale)	93% highly religious 7% religious (M = 4.28; SD = 0.512)
"I have some experience in interacting with persons suffering from depressive disorders." (multiple answers possible)	44% in my family 84% friends and acquaintances 40% in my church congregation 11% job related 2% not at all
"I'm already familiar with depressive disorders."	3.5% not at all 15.8% rather not 36.8% a bit 29.8% rather true 14.0% very much true
"In this course, I learned something new about depression."	33.3% rather not 25.0% a bit 33.3% rather true 8.3% very much true

The volunteers engaged in a pastoral care setting in their congregation were mostly female. This is comparable to other studies with volunteers in a congregation.[2] Surprisingly, the participants were about middle-aged, which is not self-

2 E.g. the data of the 5th survey of the Evangelical Church in Germany (EKD) on church-membership. The statistic distribution depends on the area of engagement. Cf. EKD, ed., *Engagement und Indifferenz. Kirchenmitgliedschaft als soziale Praxis. V. EKD-Erhebung über Kirchenmitgliedschaft* (Hannover 2014), 124. Cf. for all areas of engagement: Julia Simonson,

evident: In other contexts, many volunteers are older. The majority are highly associated with their church in general. Nearly all of them are highly religious and therefore, we can assume that religion plays an important role in their lives.

The majority of the participants already had some understanding about depression (43.8% true and rather true). Therefore, nearly half of the course participants expressed that they did not learn many new things about depression. This might be the case, as 84% had depressive friends or acquaintances, 44% experienced depression in family contexts. We, therefore, can assume that there was a high interest not only in the content of the course but also to learn more about how to deal with depression as a personal motivation. To understand more about the motivation of people who engage in voluntary work in their congregations, we explicitly asked about their motives to do so.

2.2.1 Motivation to Volunteer in the Project on Depression

Having a first look at the data, it is obvious that the most important motives are to learn more about depression, to better cope with the illness of others and to help them (Figure 1).

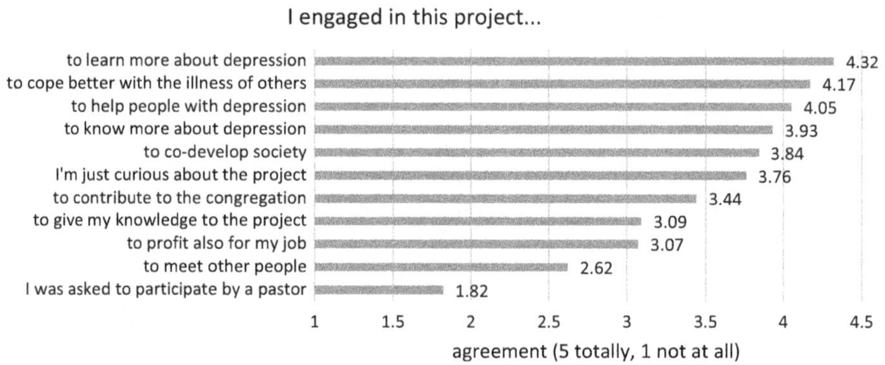

Figure 1: Motivation to engage in the project.

The less specific motives did not meet with much agreement. Only a few people were involved in this project out of a purely extrinsic motivation, for example, because their pastor asked them to do so. To know more about the structure of

Claudia Vogel and Clemens Tesch-Römer, eds., *Tabellenanhang. Freiwilliges Engagement in Deutschland – Der Deutsche Freiwilligensurvey 2014* (Wiesbaden: Springer VS, 2016), 137.

motives, a factor analysis was conducted with all project volunteers. Three main factors were identified (varimax rotation, 55% explained variance[3]) (Table 2).

Table 2: Factor analysis for motives to volunteer in the project.

Rotated component matrix[a]				
Item	**What was your motivation to participate in the project?**	**component**		
		factor 1	**factor 2**	**factor 3**
M7	I want to help people with depression	**0.686**		0.250
M9	I'm just curious about the project	**0.656**		
M10	I'd like to co-develop society with a small contribute	**0.579**		0.227
M6	I think, I can profit from the project also for my job	**0.561**	0.349	
M1	I want to meet like-minded people	**0.546**		−0.296
M5	I'd like to contribute to the project with my expertise		**0.761**	−0.248
M4	I'd like to enhance my knowledge about pastoral care	−0.257	**0.744**	0.436
M2	I'd like to contribute to the church congregation	0.209	**0.743**	−0.279
M3	I want to know more about depression			**0.717**
M11	I'm looking for possibilities to cope with the illness of others	0.366		**0.713**
M8	My pastor asked me to participate in this project		0.277	**−0.624**
	Method of extraction: main component analysis. Missing values replaced with mean method of rotation varimax with Kaisers normal distribution			

[a]rotation with 7 iterations.

Factor 1 is a combination of altruistic motivation (e.g. to develop society, to help others) with a more general motivation and a curiosity about the project ("altruism and curiosity"). The interest to meet similar people is also a part (conviviality). Factor 2 combines an altruistic motivation that includes the wish to bring one's own expert knowledge to benefit the project. The already existing competence from the professional background is brought into the project with the interest to enhance it ("contribute and learn"). Factor 3 contains a specific motivation to know more about depression in general and to cope with it ("interest in

3 This small portion of explained variance is due to the small number of participants. Listwise rotation only brought small nonsignificant changes to the factor analysis.

depression"). According to the three factors of motivation, a cluster analysis[4] identified four groups of volunteers bringing their different motivation structure to the project (Table 3).

Table 3: Cluster analysis based on 3 factors of motivation.

Cluster Analysis with Seuclid/Ward Method (n = 57, rmv)				
Ward Method		**"altruism and curiosity"**	**"contribute and learn"**	**"interested in depression"**
Cluster 1: interested in learning about depression	mean	−0.74	−0.15	0.30
	N	21.00	21.00	21.00
	SD	0.900	0.588	0.536
Cluster 2: interested experts	mean	0.48	0.91	0.61
	N	17.00	17.00	17.00
	SD	0.628	0.630	0.523
Cluster 3: interested in general	mean	−0.07	0.02	−1.74
	N	11.00	11.00	11.00
	SD	0.743	0.760	0.422
Cluster 4: interested without expert knowledge	mean	1.00	−1.57	0.31
	N	8.00	8.00	8.00
	SD	0.809	0.640	0.517
	N	57	57	57
ANOVA (all)	**Eta**	**0.646**	**0.78**	**0.868**
	Sig.	<0.001	<0.001	<0.001

The cluster analysis identifies four groups with different interests. There is a large number who are generally interested in the phenomenon of depression and therefore would like to know more about it (37%). Another 30% are experts from different backgrounds, mostly health professionals working in church or secular health care settings. Only 19% came without special interest in depression or pastoral care. The fourth group (14%) is interested in the project without special knowledge and has a high interest to support others. The ANOVA (Analysis of Variance) supports a good fit for the groups with a high level of homogeneity within each group.

4 Seuclid/Ward method, n=57 (2 excluded because of missing variables).

2.2.2 Attitudes toward Faith Communities and Health

The second question addresses the role of the faith community and its relationship to depression and health. The results show support for the idea that the congregation could support mental health (Table 4).

Table 4: Attitudes toward congregation and health.

Item	Faith communities have a potential to contribute to mental health *(scale: 1 = I don't agree at all, 5 = I totally agree)*	mean	SD	N
K5	Faith communities can offer support to relatives of sick people.	4.26	0.785	58
K2	Practicing faith together can contribute to health.	4.11	0.947	56
K3	Social relationships in faith communities can impact people's health positively or negatively.	3.25	0.977	56
K1	Faith communities don't have a potential to contribute to mental health. It's only the medical doctor who can help.	2.61	0.940	57

Overall, there's a high agreement with the idea that a congregation supports mental health. Volunteers are convinced that health and faith belong together and that faith can play a positive role in the lives of people suffering from mental diseases. Consequently, there is little agreement for item K1: that only a medical doctor can help and a faith community cannot. The highest level of agreement is regarding the offer of support to relatives of ill people (K5).

2.2.3 Attitudes toward Religion and Health (Religious Meaning Concepts)

A further interesting relationship between personal faith convictions and attitudes to mental health has been investigated (Table 5). A factor analysis identified three different factors. Factor 1 contains a positive approach to faith that can provide help through giving direction, guidance, help and solace in life. Volunteers give the highest acceptance to this factor and therefore mostly share a positive coping behavior. The second factor is about a passive God and considering humans to be responsible for the suffering in the world. The third factor leaves room for a negative and darker image of God, meaning that God is also able to test people and make them suffer.

Compared to the scale of centrality, it is possible to conclude that higher religious volunteers also are in higher agreement with factor 1 (significant correlation

Table 5: Attitudes toward faith and health.

Item	One's personal faith can be relevant in difficult situations of life. What is your experience in this regard? *(scale: 1 = I don't agree at all, 5 = I totally agree)*	mean	SD	N	Factor
C1	To me, faith is a source of comfort and hope.	4.25	0.739	54	1
C3	My personal faith helps me to make sense of situations that seem to be hopeless.	4.02	0.812	56	1
C4	God provides orientation for my life.	3.88	0.935	55	1
C2	Through my personal faith, I can activate my strengths and potentials.	3.87	0.818	50	1
C5	Human beings themselves are responsible for all sufferings in the world.	3.13	1.072	55	2
C8	I ask myself why God allows suffering to happen.	3.07	0.850	56	3
C9	Sometimes, God is very hard on people.	2.80	0.998	55	3

$r = 0.656$; $p < 0.001$). Accordingly, they also might have a positive access to religious coping. Older participants more often include a negative image of God in their faith (moderate correlation $r = 0.258$; $p = 0.065$). Between altruistic motivation (motivation factor 1) and faith attitudes there is also a significant relationship ($r = 0.515$; $p < 0{,}001$). This could lead to the assumption that one's own positive religious coping also motivates one to give something back by helping and supporting others.

3 The Study in Malawi

3.1 Mental Health Services in Malawi

Like in other African countries, mental health care in Malawi is centralized. For a population of about 17 million, mental health services are mainly offered in three mental hospitals located in the big cities of Mzuzu, Zomba, and Lilongwe. Therefore, the distances to access specialized mental health services are very far. The process of decentralization of mental health care which has taken place in Europe over the past decades, has just started there. The availability of human resources in Malawi is as low as it is in all countries of the African WHO region, where on an average 0.7 psychiatrists and 0.5 psychiatric nurses are available per 100.000 people. For comparison: In the European WHO region 9.9 psychiatrists and 23.2 psychiatric nurses are available for 100.000 people.[5]

Because of the long distances to access mental health services and due to the lack of human resources in mental health, it is estimated that in low income countries like Malawi, less than 25% of those in need of mental health care have access to these medical services.

Another factor contributing to the huge treatment gap is that knowledge about mental health is very low among trained health professionals. They often are unable to diagnose mental disorders like psychoses and affective disorders. Moreover, even among health professionals one can find many misconceptions about the causes of and treatment possibilities for mental disorders.[6]

As one way of improving access to mental health services in Malawi, like in other countries of the Global South, it has been recommended to integrate mental health services in community-based programmes thus bringing mental health services closer to the people.[7]

Since 2016 the German Institute for Medical Mission (DIFÄM) has supported and accompanied a mental health project of the Presbyterian Church of Malawi (CCAP Nkhoma Synod) which integrates mental health into the community-based health services of the Nkhoma Hospital in the Lilongwe District of Malawi. The project offers training for health professionals (nurses, clinical officers and medical doctors) in mental health. These trained health care workers form a mental health team going out to the communities to identify people with mental disorders and providing mental health services in the communities. As another component of the project, religious leaders, traditional authorities and volunteers in the community are sensitized and informed about mental health.

The participants in the study in Malawi were health care professionals working in institutions that are partners of DIFÄM. Some of them were involved in the mentioned mental health project. Accordingly, we did not include questions about the motivation to participate and help in a particular project. Instead, we focused on the relationship between spirituality, health and faith communities and compared these results to the German sample. The sample consists of 63 health care professionals and their attributes are shown in Table 6.

---

5 World Health Organization, *Mental Health Atlas 2017* (Geneva: World Health Organization, 2018), 33.

6 Cf. chapter II.5. in this volume: Paul Mekani and Japhet Myaba, *Mental Health and Mental Disorders: Knowledge, Perceptions and Attitudes Towards People with Mental Diseases. Results of a Quantitative and Qualitative Study Conducted in Lilongwe District, Malawi.*

7 Cf. for example: Graham Thornicroft, T. Deb and C. Henderson, "Community mental health care worldwide: current status and further developments," *World Psychiatry 15(3)* (2016): 276–286.

Table 6: Characteristics of the Malawian sample.

Characteristics	Results in Malawi (percent)
Role in the church congregation	45 health professionals (80%) 2 volunteers (4%) 9 other* (16%)
Gender	52% female, 48% male
Age	M = 30.8 years (SD = 9.37 years, min 19, max 61)
Religiosity (scale of centrality, Z-Scale)	93% highly religious 7% religious (M = 4.42; SD = 0.471)
"I have some experience in interacting with persons suffering from depressive disorders."	23% in my family 60% friends and acquaintances 18% in my church congregation 16% not at all

*Other professionals working in the health care system, e.g. human resource manager, accountant.

3.2 Results

3.2.1 The Malawian Sample

Overall, there is a high religiosity in the Malawian sample. The participants were much younger than in the German sample and there are more males than in the German sample. Fewer people in Malawi have had previous experience with depression in their personal social contexts. Only 2% in Germany had no experience with depression beforehand, in Malawi it was 16%. This might be due to the young age of the Malawian participants or because even people working in the health care system are not as aware of depression as non-health professionals in Germany.

3.2.2 Attitudes toward Church Congregation and Health

Comparing the attitudes and mind-set towards the role of the congregation to promote health, the Malawian participants rated the positive influence of congregations on health higher than the Germans (Figure 2).

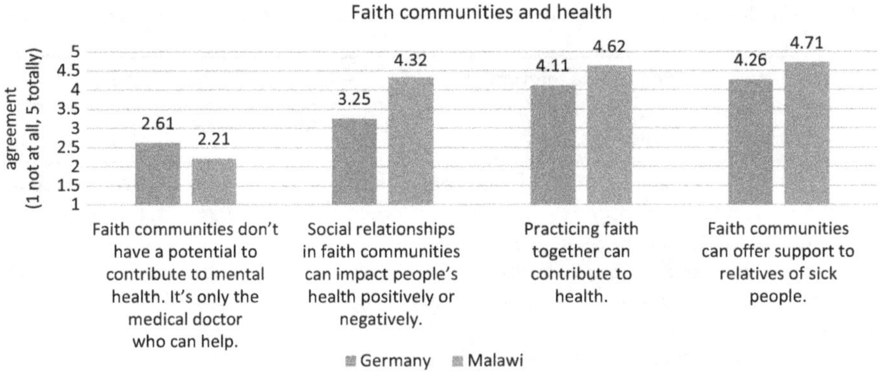

Figure 2: Comparing attitudes toward faith communities and health in Malawi and Germany.

The results show moderately higher levels of the positive impact of the congregation in the Malawian sample. All mean differences between the Malawian and the German sample are significant ($p<0.05$). Interestingly, there is an ambivalence towards the idea that only medical doctors can help. Half of the sample is convinced that only doctors can help whereas the other half denies this idea. Another interesting observation is that professionals without contact to depressed people agree more to the idea that practising faith can contribute to health. Professionals that have already experienced depression in their social context are less convinced about the supportive role of practising faith.[8] This could mean that people who have had experience with depression share a more realistic view of the relationship between religion and health in the sense that religion could support health but that this is no guarantee for a better mental health. In short: There is no causal relationship between practising faith (e.g. prayer, attending services) and health; people who pray can also become depressed.

3.2.3 Attitudes toward Religion and Health (Religious Meaning Concepts)

Surprisingly, we found nearly the same factor structure in questions about religion and health. As in the German study, three different factors can be distinguished. Compared to the German sample, the Malawian participants agree significantly more to the positive contribution of the community to mental health (Table 7).

8 All 16% that had no contact with depressive patients beforehand rated item K2 as rather or fully agree. 21% of the professionals that had contact before rated this as not at all or rather not true.

Table 7: Attitudes toward religion and health in Malawi and Germany.

Item	*One's personal faith can be relevant in difficult situations of life. What is your experience in this regard?*	Germany		Malawi		
		mean	SD	mean	SD	p-value
C1	To me, faith is a source of comfort and hope.	4.25	0.739	4.75	0.507	p < *0.001*
C3	My personal faith helps me to make sense of situations that seem to be hopeless.	4.02	0.812	4.34	1.173	*n.s.*
C4	God provides orientation for my life.	3.88	0.935	4.86	0.353	p < *0.001*
C2	Through my personal faith, I can activate my strengths and potentials.	3.87	0.818	4.64	0.731	p < *0.001*
C5	Human beings themselves are responsible for all sufferings in the world.	3.13	1.072	1.85	1.353	p < *0.001*
C8	I ask myself why God allows suffering to happen.	3.07	0.850	3.39	1.429	*n.s.*
C9	Sometimes, God is very hard on people.	2.80	0.998	1.97	1.426	p < *0.001*

The results were mostly comparable in size and effect. One item showed a difference: that of humans being responsible for all suffering in the world (p < *0.001*). In Germany, there is a moderate agreement to this interpretation of the theodicy, whereas Malawian health care professionals mostly rate this as rather not true. However, the results can be interpreted as a stronger religious orientation system in the Malawian cultural context that relies on a positive influence of God in someone's life (C1, C2, C4). The German sample agreed significantly less to these items. This idea can be supported with the correlation analysis of personal faith with the score of centrality. People with a higher score of centrality tend to rate the items about theodicy lower than less religious individuals (C7: $r = -0.305$, $p < 0.05$; C8: $r = -0.355$, $p < 0.05$).

4 Some Conclusions

Sample differences: Comparing both samples, Malawian participants are of a lower age which reflects the difference in the medium age in Malawi (30.8 years) and in Germany (46.8 years).[9] The volunteers in the German sample are

9 Source: Wikipedia article, *Liste der Länder der Welt nach Lebensaltermedian*, in URL: https://de.wikipedia.org/wiki/Liste_der_Länder_der_Welt_nach_Lebensaltermedian (last accessed on 1 April 2020).

mostly females. Religiosity is nearly the same in both samples, a little higher in Malawi (Germany: 4.28 / Malawi: 4.42).

Experience with depression: In Malawi less participants have experience with depression than in Germany. This is striking as the Malawian participants are mostly health professionals whereas the Germans are non-professionals. Though there are no reliable figures about the prevalence of depression in Malawi, this difference might be due to a lower prevalence of depression among the Malawian population. Another factor might be that depression and its symptoms, even among health professionals, are not as well known in Malawi, while in Germany people have been sensitized about the disease over the past years. For example, the media has drawn a lot of attention to depression and burnout, not only but also in connection with suicides of well-known persons, like the football player Robert Enke (Hannover 96) in 2009.

Attitudes toward faith and health: Most of the volunteers in Germany and health professionals in Malawi share a positive interpretation of the relation between their faith community and their impact on health. Both groups are convinced religion and health are somehow rather positively related. In their opinion, mental health can be supported by the help of a religious congregation through social cohesion and practising of faith itself. Concerning the motivation to volunteer, the German participants tend to actively engage in the congregation to share their religious convictions. This might be according to their highly religious worldview and mind-set. As religion plays a central role in their lives, they like to share this view as a resource with others. In the Malawian sample, the centrality of religion is even higher, as is the agreement to the significance of a supporting religious congregation. This significant difference may also relate to the differences in the health system and therefore the importance of additional social and religious support of the congregation.

The role of medical doctors: Among the Malawian participants, more are convinced that the medical doctor alone can heal than among the Germans. This phenomenon might be due to the sample difference. Health professionals in Malawi have a very high regard for the medical system. They often overestimate the role of medicine as opposed to therapeutic approaches of traditional medicine and faith-healers which are still very common in Malawi. On the contrary, more and more people in Germany are critical of the one-dimensional medical approach to health and healing which is still prevalent in the German context.

Cultural differences in faith as religious orientation: In Germany, also negative sides of one's religion, such as God's testing or punishment and suffering in the world are much more common than in Malawi. Malawian participants tend to interpret faith in an exclusively positive way. This reflects the positive attitude towards religion in general and Christianity in particular in Malawi where about 80% of the population are Christians. Malawian people usually have a very strong relationship to God. God is perceived as the Sustainer of one's life and the Saviour in difficult circumstances.

Motivation to serve as volunteers in the German sample: The results show that most of the volunteers do not engage only for personal reasons, but are mixing altruistic, job-related and personal motives. The high level of those who are genuinely interested in depression can be explained with the setting of a pastoral care training about depression. Surprisingly, there are a respectable number of volunteers with an expert background, who would like to share their knowledge for the benefit of the project, according to an altruistic motive. They also hope to learn something from the project that they can use for their job. Thus, it could be a win-win-situation to implement such projects in church communities.

Paul Mekani and Japhet Myaba

Mental Health and Mental Disorders: Knowledge, Perceptions, and Attitudes towards People with Mental Diseases

Results of a Quantitative and Qualitative Study Conducted in Lilongwe District, Malawi

1 Introduction

Health systems have not yet adequately responded to the global burden of mental disorders. As a consequence, the gap between the need for treatment and its provision is large all over the world. In low-income and middle-income countries, between 76 and 85 per cent of people with severe mental disorders receive no treatment for their disorder; the corresponding range for high-income countries is also high: between 35 per cent and 50 per cent.[1]

According to Alem, Jacobsson and Hanlon, in Western countries, community-based mental health services have become the preferred model for delivery of psychiatric care, in contrast to the more traditional mental hospital-based services.[2] In the Western setting, the different elements of a community-based service are well-recognized and include downsizing mental hospitals, the establishment of psychiatric units in general hospitals and the formation of community-based mental health teams.[3]

However, in most African countries the progress towards community mental health care is still hampered by a lack of resources, with specialist psychiatric care essentially based in large, centrally located mental hospitals.[4] In Malawi, mental health services are centralized in three units which are each located in one of the three regions of Malawi. This means that most people with mental

---

1 Cf. World Health Organisation: *Mental Health Action Plan 2013–2020* (2014), 8; in URL: http://apps.who.int/iris/bitstream/10665/89966/1/9789241506021_eng.pdf?ua=1 (last accessed on 1 April 2020).

2 Cf. Atalay Alem, Lars Jacobsson and Charlotte Hanlon, "Community-based mental health care in Africa: mental health workers' views," *Journal of World Psychiatry* 7(1) (2008): 54.

3 Alem, et al., "Community-based mental health care in Africa," 54.

4 Cf. Felix Kauye, Rachel Jenkins and Atif Rahman, "Training primary health care workers in mental health and its impact on diagnosis of common mental disorders in primary care of a developing country, Malawi: a cluster-randomized controlled trial," *Psychological Medicine* 44(3) (2014): 657–666.

https://doi.org/10.1515/9783110674217-009

health problems do not get help early as they have to be referred or travel long distances to a mental hospital. In a study done in Malawi, Kauye et al. noted severe shortages of mental health professionals in the country, and concluded that integration of mental health into existing primary and community health services is the most feasible way of increasing access to services for people with mental health problems.[5]

A study conducted in Malawi reported that 28.8 per cent of patients attending primary health care services have common mental health problems like depression or anxiety.[6] A similar study conducted by the World Health Organization (WHO) in 2002 noted depression to be the fourth leading cause of disability in Malawi, after HIV, cataracts, and malaria.[7]

The Nkhoma Hospital, a mission hospital owned by the Presbyterian Church,[8] is situated on the edge of Lilongwe District and bordering on the Dedza District in Malawi. It has a 250 bed-capacity and serves a population of about 378,000 people. It is the primary referral hospital for the surrounding nine government health centres. Due to its location, the hospital gets an influx of patients seeking good specialist care from both districts as well as the neighbouring countries of Mozambique and Zambia. Apart from offering general health services, patients with mental health disorders are treated.

From June 2014 to March 2015, the Nkhoma Hospital out-patient department registered 50 patients with diagnoses of psychosis and more than 300 with epilepsy (Nkhoma Hospital Registry, 2015). Some of them were admitted to the medical wards for treatment of mental disorders. Severe cases were referred to the Bwaila Psychiatric Unit, a specialized mental hospital in the central region of Malawi, for further treatment.

However, follow-up care of patients in the community has always been difficult. Most of them do not come back for review until they have a relapse. The lack of follow-up care by the hospital is due to lack of funding and proper follow-up structures in mental health care services.

The present study was conducted to analyze the status of mental health care services in the Nkhoma Hospital catchment area and to propose the options of integrating mental health services within the hospital's existing primary health care services.

---

5 Cf. Felix Kauye et al., "Increasing the capacity of health surveillance assistants in community mental health care in a developing country, Malawi," *Malawi Medical Journal* 23(3) (2011): 85.

6 Cf. Kauye et al., "Training primary health care workers,"657–666.

7 Cameron Bowie, "The burden of diseases in Malawi," *Malawi Medical Journal* 18 (3) (2006): 103–110.

8 Church of Central Africa Presbyterian – Nkhoma Synod.

The specific objectives were:

- To establish an overview of the knowledge about mental health and mental disorders among health professionals and non-professionals.
- To investigate the perception of community members towards people with mental disorders.
- To explore the status of mental health service delivery at the Nkhoma Hospital and its catchment area.

The situational analysis was a cross-sectional study which used mixed methods in both data collection and analysis. Survey strategy was used to gain an overall picture, and a more detailed analysis was achieved through specific case studies within the targeted population. Throughout the situation analysis, a deductive approach was adopted to achieve the set objectives.

Ethical approval to conduct the study was obtained from the National Health Sciences Research Committee of the Ministry of Health. Authorization was obtained from the Medical Director of Nkhoma Mission Hospital to conduct the study.

2 Quantitative Study

2.1 Methodology

The participants in the quantitative study comprised nurses, clinical officers, medical doctors, medical assistants, community health workers (in Malawi known as Health Surveillance Assistants, HSAs), hospital chaplains and community members.[9] We failed to find patients with mental disorders during the time of data collection. All participants included in the survey were older than 18 years.

The total number of participants was 208. Among these were 111 health workers and 97 community members. There were two questionnaires, one for the health workers and the other one for the community members. These questionnaires were different in some aspects. For instance, the questionnaire for the health workers was designed in a way to capture their knowledge of the management of mental health problems in general.

Data management and analysis were performed with use of Statistical Package for Social Sciences (SPSS) version 16.0. Plausibility checks were

9 Health workers and community members who participated in the study had different questionnaires.

performed to assess the quality of data concerning completeness, rightness and consistency. The study used descriptive statistics with frequency distribution tables and figures. Inferential analysis using Chi-Square test was applied to test for strength of association between dependent variables (e.g. depression) and the independent variables (e.g. physical and sexual violence). The significance of association was determined at a significance level of 0.05 (two-tailed).

2.2 Key Findings: Health Workers

2.2.1 Description of the Sample

The health workers (n=111) who participated in the survey were from the Nkhoma Hospital and from six health centres in the hospital catchment area. The majority of them (61.3 %) were males.

The participants who were all 20 years or older were categorized into four age groups: <20 years, 20–29 years, 30–40 years, and >40 years. Majority of the participants (49 %) were of age range 30–40 years.

2.2.2 Education and Profession

As shown in Figure 1, more than half of the health workers (64.2 %) had achieved a secondary education level.

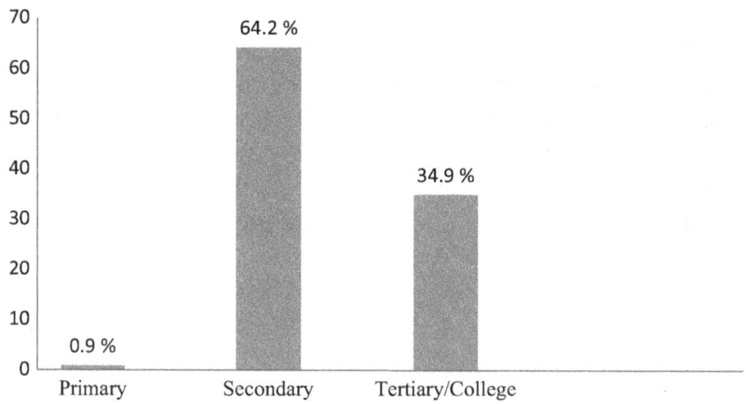

Figure 1: Education levels of participants.

The majority of the health workers were community health workers (66.7 %) who work in the rural community setting (Table 1).

Table 1: Profession of health workers.

Cadre	Frequency	Percentage
Clinical officers	4	3.6
Community health workers	74	66.7
Medical assistants	3	2.7
Nurses	24	21.6
Medical doctors	2	1.8
Others	4	3.6
Total	111	100.0

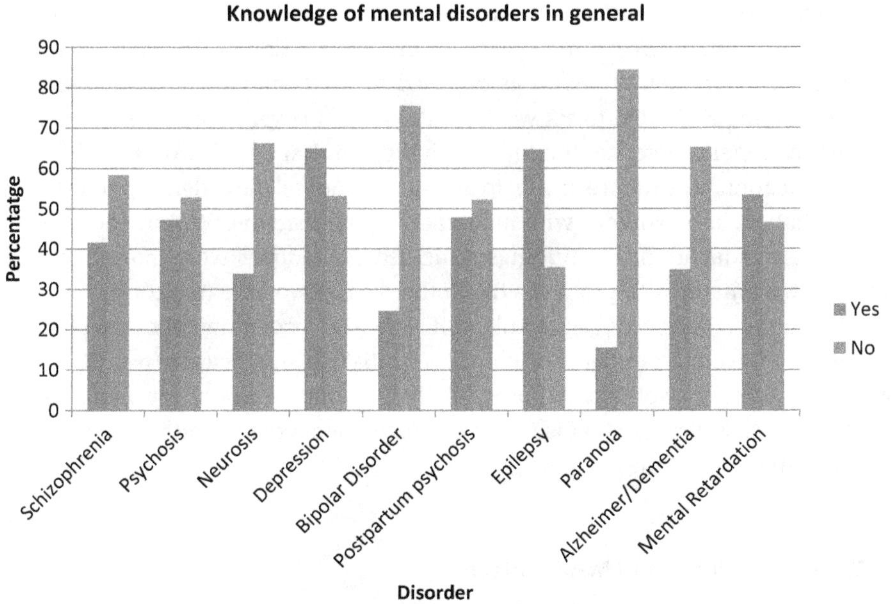

Figure 2: Knowledge of mental health disorders.

2.2.3 Knowledge on Mental Disorders in General

The majority of health workers had very poor knowledge of mental health and mental disorders. For instance, one community health worker defined mental health as "a problem of the brain". Participants were asked if they were able to identify people suffering from a particular disorder. The results are presented in the figure below.

Most participants (>50 %) could not identify a particular type of illness apart from a general recognition of mental diseases, such as depression, epilepsy, and mental retardation.

The symptoms or characteristics which participants often mentioned were in the category of disorganized behavior, and reduced level of functioning. This, therefore, indicates that those clients with unspecific symptoms such as social isolation, quietness, and reduced self-care would not be identified as early as possible for prompt management. Given such symptoms, clients would not be taken to the hospital because they are not causing problems to the community.

When results were cross-tabulated between recognition of mental disorders and occupation, there was a significant relationship between occupation of health workers and recognition of mental disorders (p=0.000). Those with a tertiary education included nurses and clinicians who had undergone a prescribed training program of two or three years. During their training, they had attended a basic course in mental health as opposed to the community health workers whose training is limited to six weeks and does not cover mental health. Given this educational difference, the findings indicated that health workers with tertiary education were more likely to recognize mental disorders amongst patients than health workers without tertiary qualifications. Within those who had tertiary education, the findings indicated that nurses were more likely to recognize mental health problems than other health workers (p=0.000).

When the results between the place of work and recognition of mental health disorders were cross-tabulated, there was a statistical significance (p=0.00) indicating that health workers stationed at the Nkhoma Hospital are more likely (69.9%) to recognize mental diseases amongst patients than health workers from the surrounding facilities.

2.2.4 Factors Related to Mental Disorder

The majority of health workers were able to identify factors that can predict mental health problems or are related with mental problems (see Figure 3). The most highly scored factor was drug and alcohol abuse (88.5 %).

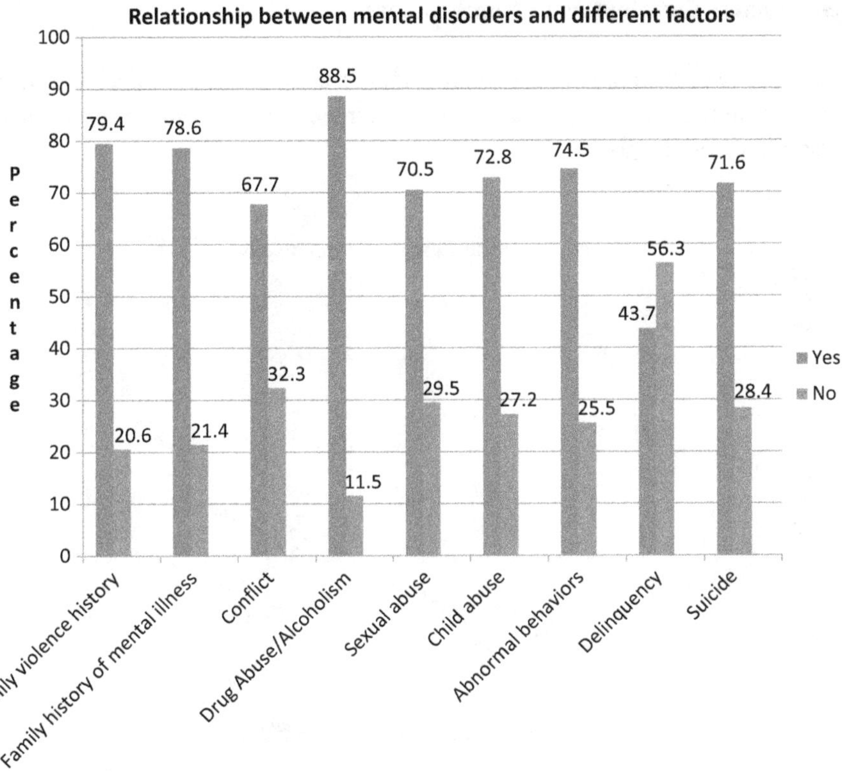

Figure 3: Factors that are related to mental disorders.

Suicide and delinquency were also reported as factors related to mental disorders although they are well known to be consequences of primary mental disorders.

2.3 Key Findings: Community Members

2.3.1 Description of the Sample

The majority of the community participants were females (67.7%). The majority (39.1%) of the participants were of the age category 40 years and above.

2.3.2 Factors Contributing to Mental Disease

The majority of the community members (88.3%) agreed that magic can precipitate mental health problems. In Figure 4, percentages represent proportions of respondents per response.

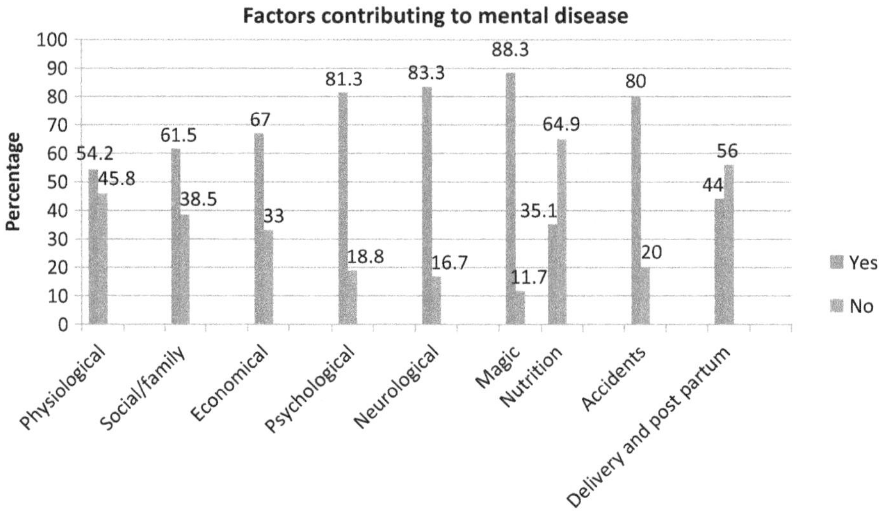

Figure 4: Factors contributing to mental disease.

2.3.3 Treatment Options

Participants were asked about the effectiveness of different treatment options. Their answers are listed in Figure 5. Majority of the participants (95.8 %) indicated that modern medication was helpful in the treatment of mental health problems.

2.4 Health Facilities

The Nkhoma Hospital is surrounded by 9 health centres. Out of these health centres, 8 refer their patients directly to the Nkhoma Hospital for further treatment. The survey included 6 of the 9 health centres. A nurse or clinician on duty during data collection responded to the questionnaire.

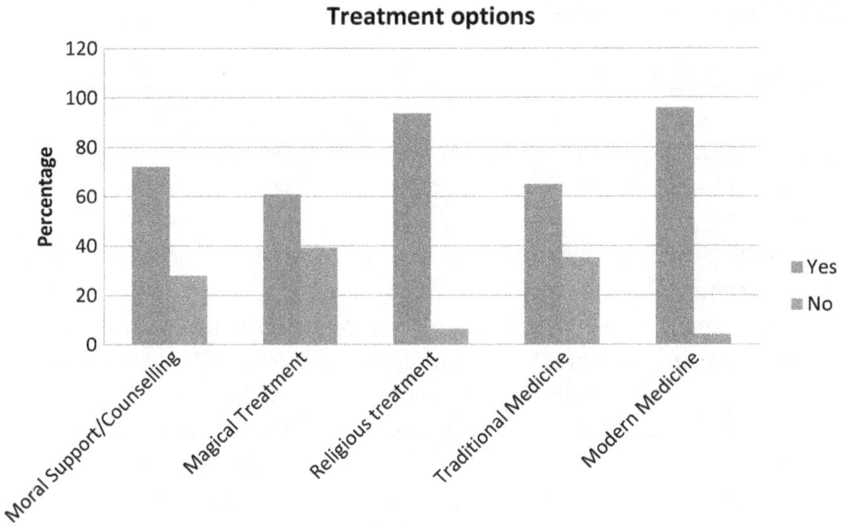

Figure 5: Treatment options.

2.4.1 Availability of Drugs

The findings of the survey showed that all the health facilities enrolled in the study do not have adequate psychotropic drugs. Some of the antipsychotic drugs available at the Nkhoma Hospital are taken from the Bwaila Psychiatric Unit. The availability of anticonvulsants in all the health facilities is due to epilepsy clinics conducted in these health facilities which receive free drugs from the government although they are not always in stock.

2.4.2 Records of Patients

Most of the health facilities (66 %) do not have records of patients admitted and referred to any hospital. Therefore, the assumption is that mental health services are not offered. One of the health facilities with records of patients with mental disorders is the Nkhoma Hospital.

3 Qualitative Study

3.1 Methodology

The participants in this study were health workers (nurses, clinicians and community health workers), key community members, and clients who were with their guardians.

The participants were purposively selected. The study included 5 focus group discussions of 6 to 12 participants in each session: One of these included 10 clients with mental health problems who were mentally stable, one with 10 guardians of persons with mental health problems, one with 9 key community members (police officers, village chiefs, teachers, counselors), two with health workers. The 18 participating health workers were divided into groups of medical personnel (nurses and clinicians) and a group of community health workers. In-depth interviews were done until data saturation was achieved.

Qualitative data were analyzed using content analysis in which themes and subthemes were derived from the narratives of the stories. It also involved transcribing the recorded data, coding and document analysis of secondary data.

3.2 Definitions of Mental Health and Mental Disorders

When health workers were asked about "What is mental health", one of the health workers defined mental health as "psychological, emotional and mental well-being of an individual which makes someone to function in an optimal way."

The guardians defined it as "a state whereby an individual is able to function properly", while one of the clients said that "mental health is when someone is able to do things well on his own."

These statements indicated some knowledge when compared to a WHO definition of mental health which refers to mental well-being as our emotions, our thoughts and feelings, our ability to solve problems and overcome difficulties, our social connection, and our understanding of the world around us.[10]

As to mental disorders, health workers said mental health problems were conditions "when an individual fails to behave himself properly in the society." Others mentioned "an abnormal behavior like picking up rubbish, undressing in public."

---

10 Cf. Silvana Galderisi et al., "Toward a new definition of mental health," *World Psychiatry* 14(2) (2015): 231–233; in URL: http://doi.org/10.1002/wps.20231 (last accessed on 1 April 2020).

The guardians in their own understanding said, "When an individual is acting abnormally such as running away from home, it is a mental health problem." They also stated that, "Sometimes a person starts with fainting or convulsing, and then later behaves abnormally. When the person is asked what happened, he does not know what happened to him."

A client and her guardian described a mental health problem as a condition "when a person has so many problems. Such a person does things or acts in a disturbed manner". Some of the examples they mentioned were "beating up people", "refusing to breastfeed their own children and undressing", "being unable to do things that a person who is well can do."

Instead of defining mental disorders, one of the community members gave an example and said: "If you dress him up, he undresses, he runs away, throws away food; if he is tied up he unties himself and runs away … When this happens we say that the person has mental illness."

These are some of the examples of the responses or explanations that guardians used to explain the symptoms: "When we talk to him, he responds by talking totally different things from what you talked about … "; "He is disturbed, we do not agree on what to do, we just see that someone has become mad … ."

Undressing in public, laughing out of place, and beating up others were also some of the symptoms that were reported by most respondents as common symptoms of mental health disorders.

The definitions of mental disorders and descriptions of people suffering from mental diseases given by the participants show that they mainly concentrated on talking about the behaviour of people affected by mental disorders. According to WHO, mental disease is a disease that affects the way people think, feel, behave, or interact with others.[11] This, therefore, indicates that participants had some knowledge but they still need to understand the concept better. Only if they understand the concept properly, health workers will be able to manage mental disorders properly.

3.3 Assumptions about the Conditions Underlying Mental Diseases

In the group of health workers, mental disorders were described as a condition which comes due to medical or social problems. As an example, they referred

11 Cf. Galderisi et al., "Toward a new definition of mental health," 231–233; in URL: http://doi.org/10.1002/wps.20231 (last accessed on 1 April 2020).

to depression developing after losing loved ones. Some health workers referred to it as "madness" which is a discriminating expression. Others reported that a person with a mental disorder acts abnormally, deviating from what is expected from the normal behavior in the community. However, health workers reported that mental disorders could also be a result of bewitchment or magic.

On the same level, guardians' descriptions were not far from what was said by the health workers. They described mental disorders as when someone has become insane or is indeed mad.

Another respondent from the group of community members said: "The kinds of mental disorders are known according to the cause of the disease such as smoking chamba[12] and abusing alcohol." For example, it was said that "if someone has been smoking chamba for a long time, later the person develops a mental disease; the person becomes very talkative, picks up rubbish and beats up people."

One of the clients and her guardian said that when a person has a mental disorder, it means that his brain or head is not functioning properly, he behaves inappropriately and does things or acts differently from other people's expectations. They further said that some people say that a mental disorder means that someone's brain has been mixed with blood, or they have a high blood pressure.

3.4 Knowledge about Specific Mental Disorders

The nurses and clinicians expressed some knowledge about specific mental disorders by saying:
- Delirium – shakes vigorously.
- Schizophrenia – at times someone is aggressive, has hallucinations.
- Mania – a person is restless, aggressive, talkative.
- Depression – the person is out of activity, does not participate.
- Puerperal psychosis – some may be mute, aggressive, deny their own babies.
- Psychosis – can also come due to medical conditions such as malaria, brain damage.
- Dementia – a person becomes forgetful, especially in old age
- Epilepsy – because of fits they also become mentally disabled.
- Anxiety – panic attack, restlessness, fear of unknown.

12 Chamba (Chichewa language) is the local name for cannabis.

The guardians could not mention specific mental disorders, but were able to mention some of the symptoms of mental diseases.

3.5 Behavior towards People with Mental Disorders

There are many misconceptions about people with mental disorders resulting in stigma and discrimination.

Due to the myths and stigma surrounding mental diseases, people with serious mental disorders are deterred from accessing mental health care. Different forms of stigma and discrimination were revealed during the focus group discussions.

A focus group discussion of health workers revealed that people with mental diseases are seen as hazardous: "Even while we were learning, our lecturers used to say that when dealing with mentally ill patients you should make sure that you are safe because they are viewed as hazardous to others … "

"People with mental diseases are believed to be spiritually possessed by people in the community," said one participant. Another said: "In the village those who have mental disorders due to alcohol abuse are ignored because people say it is because of their behavior unlike those who have mental diseases because they are physically sick."

Some health workers indicated that some people with mental disorders are abandoned because people do not want to be associated with those having such problems. The words used to explain mental diseases are also stigmatizing like "mad" or "abnormal".

In a group of guardians, some explained that people in the community considered those with mental disorders as useless. They further mentioned that some people with mental diseases are beaten up because people are tired of them. Others believe that when they beat them, they would stop being disorganized. "They think that by doing so [beating them] they can change for the better. But some people think that those with mental disorders are exaggerating or acting deliberately as if they are sick, so they think that by beating them up they will behave normally, but some people don't know that they have a disease."

One client and her guardian said that people with a mental disease should be called "having a mental disorder" instead of "mad" so as to give them respect instead of discriminating them.

The client herself admitted that people say a lot of things behind her back pertaining to the mental disease she had. But as they never say anything in her presence, she is not sure what they talk about. She confessed that she does not feel embarrassed or ashamed because she once had mental disease.

3.6 Can People with Mental Diseases Recover and Return to Work?

Health workers indicated that clients with mental diseases can get better with medication. Asked if people with mental diseases can recover and return to work, health workers were of the opinion that people with mental diseases could work again, though they viewed them as unpredictable. Others said that it depends on the cause of the disorders. Given examples about those with congenital problems in the brain, it was said that they cannot be expected to work again, but those with problems such as drug abuse or alcohol can recover as the cause is reversible.

Most of the participants in all groups agreed that people with mental diseases can recover from mental disorders and that they can go back to work if they get the required modern medication as the following statements show:

- Yes, they can, and they do recover with modern medication to an extent that they can go back to work. An example is my child. She is able to have a small business, she makes some doughnuts and sells them because she receives and takes treatment from this hospital.
- I observe a change in my child's behavior. Before she started taking treatment from the hospital her behavior was different; we could not understand one another, now we are able to understand each other. We also took her to bottom hospital [mental health hospital] at a certain time.
- My child reached a point where we had to tie him up because he used to run away from home and would go to the mountain. Later it is when we started taking him to the hospital, now he has completely changed such that he goes to the farm.
- My child was usually tied on both arms and legs, after taking him to the hospital he changed, now its history because he is able to farm as well.

However, it was also reported that even though some people change and are able to perform some activities and behave properly, there are people who still view them as "mad" and mock them. As a result, people become discouraged and some of them later become sick again.

3.7 Where do Patients Seek Help and Where Are They Taken?

Health workers said that people with mental disorders commonly went to hospitals, traditional healers and pastors for prayers. Where the client is taken to depends on the beliefs of their guardians, but mostly they are first taken to traditional healers and then to the hospital. One of the respondents said: “Even if one was seen smoking chamba and later develops a mental disorder, he is taken to the traditional healers as the first choice because they still believe they have been bewitched. The second choice is the hospital; third choice is to the pastors for prayers.”

The guardians had similar responses, but they differentiated by saying that “When a person is sick he is taken to the hospital first. When they are told that there is no illness it’s when they take the person to the traditional healer.” Some added by saying that, “Some take the person to the police so that he is arrested.”

3.8 Recommendations

Clinicians and nurses mentioned a number of services that they felt were required for mental health. They mentioned:

- There should be sensitization or awareness campaigns in the communities so that people can know where to take people with mental health problems. Also when patients go back home they should be supported because without support they become ill again.
- At the hospital, health workers should be continually trained on mental health so that those receiving the patients can have knowledge and be able to help people with mental health problems.
- Nurses and doctors should be able to make early diagnoses and help the patients in time.
- There is also need for follow-up care.
- Medications should be available in hospitals.
- Mental health needs a multi-sectoral approach because there are so many factors contributing to mental diseases. Therefore, social workers, medical professionals, pastors, psychologists, police, even the traditional healers should cooperate. They need to be sensitized and to get the correct information about mental diseases.
- Those who have recovered from mental diseases should be present during awareness campaigns.
- It should be registered wherever the patient is taken. This is needed because communication is poor due to lack of cooperation between traditional healers, the hospital, and health workers.

Community health workers shared similar recommendations. In one group, for instance, they suggested mental health awareness campaigns, orientation and refresher courses on mental health service delivery because “most community health workers do not have information to tell people in the community about mental health and mental health problems." They also asked if there could be a special department or ward for people with mental health problems at the Nkhoma Hospital. Moreover, they recommended a survey to be conducted in the Nkhoma communities to assess the extent and impact of mental health problems.

One of the clients and her guardian expressed their hope that people with mental diseases should be treated just as any other patient with general illness, without segregation.

4 Conclusions

4.1 Knowledge Gap

Generally, there is a knowledge gap among health workers and community members on mental health provision and related issues. It is also clear that the community members have a poor perception of people with mental health problems. Participants were able to understand that those with mental problems can become functional again. This was evident from the focus group discussions with health workers and community members as well, although they indicated that it is dependent on the prevailing factors and if the cause is dealt with.

4.2 The Role of Spirituality

The findings of the study revealed that the majority of the community members believe that mental diseases can also be a result of magic or bewitchment. In a focus group discussion of health workers, the members reported that magic or bewitchment is one of the contributing factors of mental disorders. The Nkhoma Hospital as a Mission Hospital does not support the belief in witchcraft or bewitchment. Surprisingly, some of the members from the church believe that magic can also be responsible for the cause of mental diseases. Surprisingly, even Christians believe that magic can cause mental diseases.

There are about 75 traditional healers surrounding the Nkhoma Hospital who also attend to patients with different diseases including mental disorders. The traditional healers have indicated that one of the causes of mental diseases is magic. It is in this regard that the researchers in this study thought it would be wise to include the role of spirituality in mental health issues.

According to Arrey et al., spirituality/religiosity can influence the way patients perceive health and disease, and their interaction with other people.[13] According to Malawi International Religious Freedom Report, Malawi is a predominantly Christian nation with 86 per cent of its people being Christians.[14] Church gatherings are one of the biggest source of networking. Most people seek God to intervene in the problems they have. They feel comforted in seeking God during illnesses.

Most of the patients at the Nkhoma Hospital are spiritual and open to pastoral counselling. Religious needs related to their disease can affect their mental health while failure to meet these needs may impact their quality of life. The hospital has five chaplains who offer spiritual support to patients admitted in the hospital.

However, although religion is usually portrayed as a source of comfort, individuals may also experience strain in their religious lives. Religion and spirituality can be damaging to mental health by means of negative religious coping, misunderstanding and miscommunication, and negative beliefs. For example, in Africa, and Malawi in particular, there are other church groups which do not allow their members to go to hospital when they are sick, and they do not take children to hospital for immunization.

Beliefs that diseases are a result of demons lead members to go to church for prayers to exorcise the demons. However, not every disease can be a result of demons. This might lead to a delay in seeking treatment and to complications later in life which might be difficult to reverse. Surprisingly, even Christians believe in magic and the majority of them believe that diseases are also caused by demons.

4.3 Stigma and Discrimination

Although stigmatizing attitudes are not limited to mental disorders, the public seems to disapprove of persons with psychiatric disabilities significantly more than of persons with physical illnesses.[15]

13 Cf. Agnes Ebotabe Arrey, Johan Bilsen, Patrick Lacor and Reginald Deschepper, "Spirituality/Religiosity: A Cultural and Psychological Resource among Sub-Saharan African Migrant Women with HIV/AIDS in Belgium," *PLoS ONE* 11(7) (2016); in URL: https://doi.org/10.1371/journal.pone.0159488 (last accessed on 14 May 2019).

14 Cf. Malawi International Religious Freedom Report (2014); in URL: *https://www.state.gov/documents/organization/238446.pdf* (last accessed on 1 April 2020).

15 Cf. Patrick W. Corrigan and Amy C. Watson, "Understanding the impact of stigma on people with mental illness," *World Psychiatry* 1(1) (2002): 16–20.

For people living with mental disorders, being stigmatized is as painful as the mental disorders themselves. The stigma causes society to develop the following attitudes and actions toward people with mental disorders:
- Fear
- Mistrust
- Prejudice
- Violence against those with mental disorders

The effect of stigma on people living with mental diseases causes them to develop an intense fear of 'coming out', leading to a delay in seeking necessary mental health care. In this case, the patients develop a practice of self-stigmatization and endure discrimination. This leads to their conditions becoming chronic without getting the necessary attention.

This stigma does not only affect the patients, but even their families are affected negatively. This shows that stigma and discrimination are enemies in dealing with mental diseases. There is need for mass awareness and sensitization so that these patients are accepted.

5 A Way Forward: Integration of Mental Health in Community-Based Health Services of the Nkhoma Hospital

The presented findings of the situational analysis formed a basis for the establishment of a community mental health project targeting the hospital's catchment population.

These are some of the activities implemented by the project:
- Outreach clinics were established where patients with epilepsy and mental diseases are treated close to where they live. This has reduced the costs the patients incur when accessing services at the hospital. The same outreach clinics provide antenatal and family planning services as well as under-five clinics. This helps to reduce the stigma attached to attending a mental health clinic.
- Patients who are not stable are followed up through domiciliary care (home visits). Through such visits the lives of people who attempted suicide were rescued.
- Self-help groups were established for people with substance abuse and alcoholism. Through these meetings, some clients have been identified and

referred to a mental hospital for addiction and recovery programs. So far, eight clients have undergone the addiction recovery program and are being followed up. Some of them have completely recovered while others are still recovering but also have changed tremendously.

- Alcoholics Anonymous Group. This is a group of people who were addicted to alcohol and have decided to quit abusing alcohol. They are the same people who underwent an intensive addiction recovery program.
- Meetings with guardians are held to encourage them to support the clients at home.
- Stakeholders and community leaders are invited to meetings where they learn about mental health and the project. Some of the stakeholders are the Lilongwe District Health Office, Bwaila Psychiatric Hospital, Saint John of God Mental Hospital, Ministry of Health Headquarters, World Vision and Health Centres.

Even after a short time of implementation, this project has had a positive impact on the lives of the communities as people now understand better why people with mental disorders behave differently from others.

III Approaches to Improve Mental Health

Beate Jakob

Global Mental Health

An Overview

1 Impact of Mental Disorders on the Global Burden of Diseases

Historically, mental health has not been a global health priority compared to communicable diseases and some of the major noncommunicable diseases like cardiovascular disorders and cancer.[1] In Africa, for example, health care in general has always been poorly funded and mental health in particular has received almost no attention from governments. Even today, many policy makers in other continents are of the opinion that Africa's only problems are infectious diseases and hunger. The Millennium Development Goals (MDGs) set by the United Nations to be achieved by 2015 did not include mental health directly or indirectly in their goals.

After the beginning of the new millennium things have changed to some degree. Following the World Health Report 2001: "Mental health – new understanding, new hope",[2] there has been a growing awareness of mental disorders having a major impact on global health.

Since 2011, the World Health Organization (WHO) has collected data[3] that give an alarming picture of global mental health. Mental health disorders[4] are found among all ages and across all cultures. It is estimated that about 25 percent

1 Harvey A. Whiteford et al., "Global burden of disease attributable to mental and substance use disorders: findings from the Global Burden of Disease Study 2010," in URL: www.thelancet.com, published online August 29, 2013: http://dx.doi.org/10.1016/S0140-6736(13)61611-6 (last accessed on 1 April 2020).

2 World Health Organization, "The World Health Report 2001: Mental Health: New Understanding, New Hope," *World Health Organization* (2001): 110–112.

3 All data regarding global mental health are available on the WHO website; URL: http://www.who.int/mental_health/en/ (last accessed on 1 April 2020).

4 According to the International Classification of Diseases and Related Health Problems, Tenth Revision (ICD-10) mental disorders include conditions such as depression, bipolar affective disorder, anxiety, schizophrenia and other psychoses, dementia, intellectual disabilities, conditions due to abuses of alcohol and other substances, and developmental disorders including autism. Though being neurological conditions, epilepsy and dementia are sometimes regarded as mental health conditions as they share common aspects with mental disorders in terms of the provision of services. Cf.: Movement for Global Mental Health, in URL: http://globalmentalhealth.org/node/190 (last accessed on 1 April 2020).

https://doi.org/10.1515/9783110674217-010

of all human beings suffer from a psychiatric or behavior related disease at a certain point in their life. Mental health disorders affect people of all ages, and about half of mental disorders begin before the age of 14. Between 10 and 20 percent of the world's children and adolescents have mental disorders or problems.[5] Globally, more than 300 million people of all ages suffer from depression.[6] It is estimated that 20–30 percent of patients in developing countries who visit a primary care facility suffer from one or more neuropsychiatric disorder.[7]

Mental disorders are not only causes of premature deaths, but also negatively affect the quality of life, e.g., the ability to work, to relate and to enjoy life. The WHO has tried to quantify this loss in quality of life in a term called Years Lived with Disability (YLD). Together with the reduction of life expectancy, the figure of YLD then leads to the figure of Disability Adjusted Life Years (DALYs) which is the indicator of a disease's contribution to what is called the global burden of disease (GBD).[8] Knowledge about the main contributors to the GBD is necessary information that influences prioritization of health needs and resource allocation.

Mental disorders are the leading cause, worldwide, of years lived with disability and account for a significant proportion of the total global burden of disease.[9] As a result of the Global Burden of Disease Study 2013, the WHO estimates that globally 21.2 percent of Years Lived with Disability (YLDs) are caused by disorders in the mental and behavioral disorders category which is 3–5 times greater than the disability associated with all infectious diseases that count for 6 percent of YLD.[10] Unipolar depression ranks second among the top 10 disorders contributing to the global YLDs.[11]

---

5 World Health Organization, "Child and Adolescent Mental Health," *World Health Organization*, in URL: http://www.who.int/mental_health/maternal-child/child_adolescent/en/(last accessed on 1 April 2020).

6 World Health Organization, "Depression. Fact sheet," *World Health Organization* (2020), in URL: https://www.who.int/news-room/fact-sheets/detail/depression (last accessed on 1 April 2020).

7 Wolfgang Krahl, "Mental Health in Developing Countries – Global Mental Health. 4th International Symposium 10th November 2012. Munich," *Curare 36* (2013): 144–147.

8 URL: http://www.who.int/topics/global_burden_of_disease/en/ (last accessed on 1 April 2020).

9 World Health Organization & Calouste Gulbenkian Foundation, "Improving access to and appropriate use of medicines for mental disorders," *World Health Organization* (2017), in URL: http://apps.who.int/iris/bitstream/10665/254794/1/9789241511421-eng.pdf?ua=1 (last accessed on 1 April 2020).

10 Daniel Vigo, Graham Thornicroft and Rifat Atun, "Estimating the true global burden of mental illness," *Lancet Psychiatry 3* (2016), in URL: https://www.ncbi.nlm.nih.gov/pubmed/26851330 (last accessed on 1 April 2020).

11 Data from National Institute of Mental Health, in URL: http://www.nimh.nih.gov/health/statistics/global/global-ylds-contributed-by-mental-and-behavioral-disorders.shtml (last accessed on 1 April 2020).

As a consequence of the growing awareness of the impact of mental health on the global health situation, the Sustainable Development Goals (SDGs) that the UN General Assembly adopted in 2015 include mental health. Target 3.4 requests that countries: "By 2030, reduce by one third premature mortality from noncommunicable diseases through prevention and treatment and promote mental health and well-being."

Based on these findings, the WHO frequently mentions that there is "no health without mental health."[12]

2 The Mental Health Treatment Gap

So far, health systems have not adequately responded to the challenge of mental disorders. It is estimated that in many low-income countries up to 75 percent of the people with mental disorders do not have access to the treatment they need. Mental health services are often non-existent, or based in large cities, far from the people who need them. In some of the low-income countries, even less than 10 percent of the population have access to services. With regard to psychoses, in Sub-Saharan Africa the treatment gap is estimated to exceed 90 percent.[13]

The WHO Mental Health Atlas 2017[14] contains the latest estimates of global mental health resources available to prevent and treat mental disorders. As shown in Figure 1, spending on mental health is less than 1 US dollar per person per year in African countries while European countries spend more than 20 US dollars.

In low- and middle-income countries training facilities for mental health professionals are too few to provide adequate numbers of qualified personnel. In addition, some of the well-trained specialists in low- and middle-income countries migrate to countries with higher incomes.[15] The median rate of mental health professionals ranges from less than 1 per 100.000 population in African countries to 50 per 100.000 in European countries (Figure 2).

---

12 World Health Organization, "Mental health: strengthening our response," *World Health Organization* (2018), in URL: http://www.who.int/mediacentre/factsheets/fs220/en/ (last accessed on 1 April 2020).

13 Vikram Patel and Martin Prince, "Global Mental Health: a new global health field comes of age," *JAMA 303/19* (2010): 1976–1977, 1976.

14 World Health Organization, *Mental Health Atlas 2017* (Geneva: World Health Organization, 2018).

15 Shekhar Saxena, Graham Thornicorft, Martin Knapp and Harvey Whiteford, "Global Mental Health, 2. Resources for mental health: scarcity, inequity, and inefficiency," *Lancet 370* (2007): 878–889, 881.

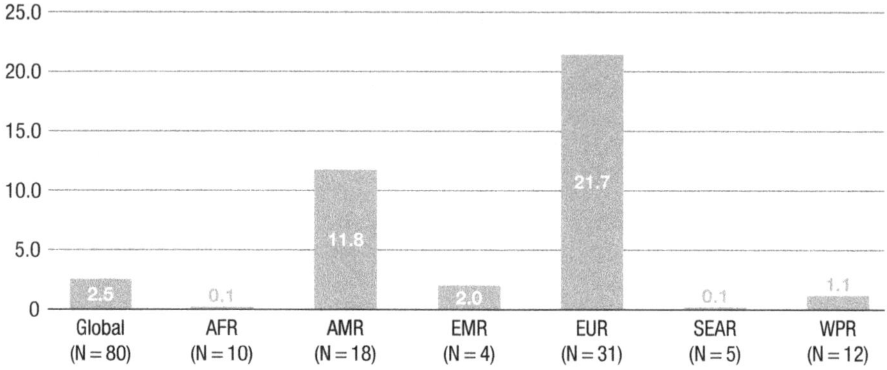

Figure 1: Government mental health expenditure per capita (US$), by WHO region Median mental health expenditure per capita, by WHO region.
Source: World Health Organization, Mental Health Atlas 2017 (Geneva: World Health Organization, 2018), 26.

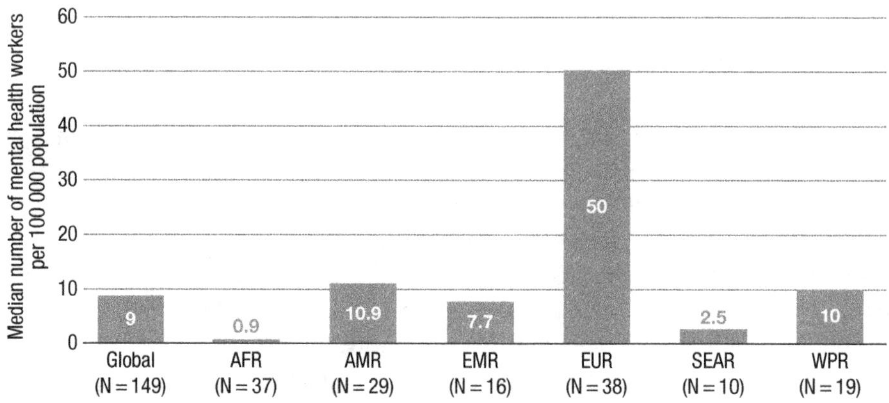

Figure 2: Medium number of mental health workers per 100 000 population, by WHO region.
Source: World Health Organization, Mental Health Atlas 2017 (Geneva: World Health Organization, 2018), 30.

According to the financial and human resouces available for treating mentally ill people, the treated prevalence of people with mental disorders (i.e. the number of people with mental disorders served by mental health services) differs significantly among the countries belonging to the various World Bank income groups: For depression the treated prevalence in high-income countries is almost 20 times higher than in low-income countries as shown in Figure 3.

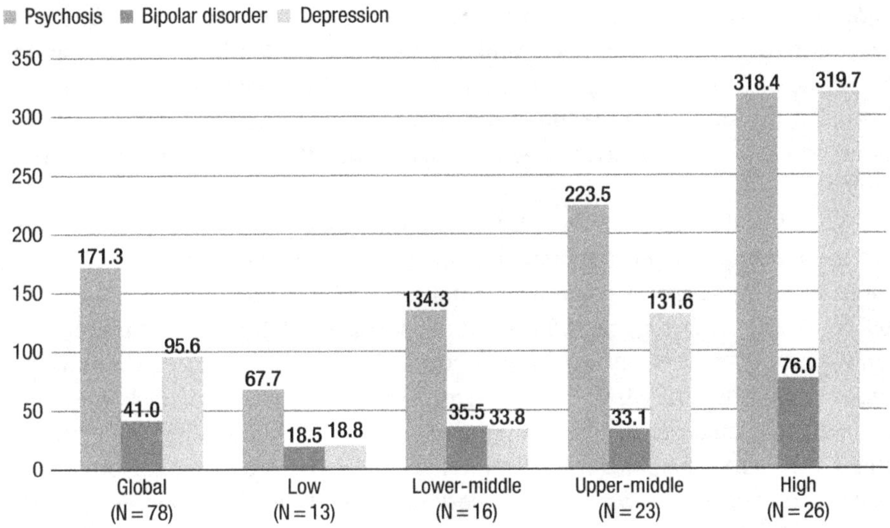

Figure 3: Total treated prevalence of psychosis, bipolar disorders and depression per 100 000 in mental health services, by World Income Group.
Source: Mental Health Atlas 2017 (Geneva: World Health Organization, 2018), 45.

3 The Need for Community-Based Mental Health Services

How can people suffering from mental disorders get access to treatment in resource limited settings? The construction of more mental health facilities can not be the only solution. There is an urgent need to bring mental health services closer to the communities where people with serious mental disorders live but do not have the chance to access quality mental health services.

Until the 19th century, all over the world the local communities were the places to deal with mental illnesses. But in the 19th century the high-income countries started to build special institutions to treat patients with mental disorders and thus isolate them from the rest of the society. This approach to treatment was later transferred to the countries of the global South.

In high-income countries, over the past decades, there has been a development towards de-institutionalizing mental health services alongside downsizing or even closing mental hospitals, building up mental health units in general hospitals, the formation of community-based mental health teams, and providing outpatient services. However, in most of the low-income countries mental health care still is provided in mental hospitals that are far away from those who are in need of treatment. 8 out of 10 psychiatric beds are located in mental hospitals, but these facilities treat only about 7 percent of all service users. These mental hospitals are often "stand-alone" institutions that are disconnected from the other levels of mental health services and of the Primary Health Care (PHC) system.

The available but often very little resources allocated to mental health care are mostly directed towards mental hospitals. Globally, 80 percent of the mental health care budget is spent for mental hospitals. In Africa, the proportion is 89 percent.[16] Accordingly, there are little resources left for community care. Only about 57 percent of all African countries have a system of community-based mental health care.[17] To give an example, in Malawi there is only one Malawian psychiatrists for the total population of about 16 million. He works in the main mental hospital in the capital. There are a good number of trained psychiatric nurses but most of them work in hospitals and offer outpatient services based at the institutions.

There is evidence that integrating mental health services into a PHC system has the best treatment results.[18] Accordingly, the WHO recommended the development of community-based mental health services by linking them to an existing PHC system and mobilizing community resources. Mental health services should be provided at the level of health centres, health posts (village clinics), and also at community level.

Ethiopia is an example of a country that is about to dezentralize its provision of mental health services. Up to the 1970s, in Ethiopia like in the other African countries there had been a consensus that improving mental health services just meant putting up more mental hospitals. In 1984 a big mental hospital was planned to be build on the outskirt of Addis Ababa, in addition to the existing mental hospital in the capital. However, at that time WHO promoted the concept of decentralization of health services according to the concept of PHC that had been promoted in 1978. Therefore, the then Director of the WHO Mental Health Division advised the Ethiopian Ministry of Health to bring the services to the regions through training mid-level health workers instead of investing all available financial resources towards a new hospital. Accordingly,

16 World Health Organization, "Mental health systems in selected low- and middle-income countries: a WHO-AIMS cross-national analysis," *World Health Organization* (2009): 61.

17 Charlotte Hanlon, Dawit Wondimagegn and Atalay Alem, "Lessons learnt in developing community mental health care in Africa," *World Psychiatry* 9 (2010): 185–189, 185.

18 Saeed Farooq, "Collaborative care for depression: a literature review and a model for implementation in developing countries," *Int Health* 5,1 (2013): 24–28.

the plan to build the hospital was given up and the training of psychiatric nurses was started. Thus mental services were being expanded to 36 regional and district hospitals where mental health care units were established. Each of these units is run by two psychiatric nurses.[19] Up to today, 450 psychiatric nurses have been trained and deployed to health facilities in Ethiopia. Nevertheless, mental health is one of the most disadvantaged health programmes in Ethiopia, both in terms of facilities and trained staff. But Ethiopia's current Mental Health Strategy aims to further develop mental health services that are decentralized and integrated at the primary level of healthcare.[20]

Where community-based mental health services exist, they still face major challenges. Much of the care is provided by primary care workers with very little training. Even if qualified personnel is available in PHC settings, due to time pressure and a predominant biomedical model of care they often reduce their services to dispensing medication. In some countries, community-based volunteers have been trained to follow up the patients and to cooperate with the health professionels. However, it is known that it is difficult to retain them without remuneration.[21]

In the following chapters, two examples of including communities in promoting mental health at local level in India and in Germany will be presented.

19 Atalay Alem, "Community-based vs. hospital-based mental health care: the case of Africa," *World Psychiatry* 1:2 (June 2002): 98–99.

20 Information from WHO, in URL: https://www.mhinnovation.net/resources/national-mental-health-strategy-ethiopia (last accessed on 1 April 2020).

21 Hanlon et al., "Lessons learnt in mental health care," 185–189, 185.

Beate Jakob

Promoting Mental Health at a Congregational Level

A Pilot Project in Germany

1 Background

Since 1906 the German Institute for Medical Mission (Deutsches Institut für Ärztliche Mission e.V./DIFÄM) has been engaged in promoting Christian health services in the countries of the Global South. In cooperation with local Christian churches and by actively involving communities, access to quality healthcare for people in resource limited settings has been improved. For more than 100 years, medical mission in general and the work of DIFÄM in particular has been understood as being confined to implementing activities in countries of the Global South.

In 2012 DIFÄM started to implement mental health projects in Germany. In partnership with the Department for Practical Theology III of the Faculty of Protestant Theology, University of Tübingen, and in cooperation with health professionals who formed an "Alliance against Depression" ("Bündnis gegen Depression"), a pilot project on "Congregations and Mental Health" which was to be implemented in Protestant congregations in Germany was planned.

What motivated a medical mission organization that so far had been focusing on improving health services in resource limited settings to be involved in such a project in Germany where most people still have access to a very high standard of healthcare? There were above all two considerations that led to DIFÄM's engagement in such a project. First, as promoting Christian health services with a focus on community-based healthcare, DIFÄM encourages European congregations to rediscover their role in health and healing and become active partners of the formal health sector. This is because the past decades have clearly revealed the deficits of the German health system dominated by a costly technical approach to health, especially in an ageing society. Second, there is a window of opportunity to introduce experiences of DIFÄM's work with communities of the Global South in Germany where many people are disappointed by a purely biomedical approach to health. In their

https://doi.org/10.1515/9783110674217-011

search for health and wholeness, people are open to approaches including the social and spiritual dimension of healing.

Why a project on depression? Depression was not only selected because in Germany the number of people suffering from depression has increased constantly over the past decades, but also because depression is a disease that affects a person as a whole. Of course, this is true for each disease. Even a broken leg has implications beyond the physical dimension. But it is especially true for depression as this disease deeply affects the person's relationship to him- or herself, to fellow human beings and also and often particularly to God. The research question of the project was: "How can congregations in their capacity as social networks and places of worship assist people suffering from depression?"

The definition of "depression" used in the project does not end with the diagnostic classification system but takes into account a wider phenomenal domain. However, in dealing with this topic, people are made aware that there is a difference between "depression" in the sense of an illness which severely affects people for a longer period on the one side, and the condition of being in a depressed mood which everybody experiences from time to time.

2 Aim and Objectives

The project was designed with the aim to make congregations aware of their health-related assets that can complement professional approaches to health, and to stimulate a process whereby these resources are activated in order to assist persons affected by depression and their relatives.

The specific objectives were:

- To create awareness about depression and to provide information about the disease and its impact on the lives of people suffering from depression and their relatives.
- To build up capacity among pastors and congregation members to interact with people suffering from depression and to offer them counselling.
- To establish links between the congregation and the professional health providers.

3 Development of Resource Materials for Congregations

The project was implemented in stages and started with field research. Quantitative and qualitative interviews were performed with people suffering from depression and their relatives, with volunteers and pastors in congregations, and with health professionals.

Based on these interviews, the project team together with health professionals of the "Alliance against Depression" developed resources (background information and tools for practical use) to be used by volunteers and pastors in congregations. The tools were tested in two congregations, adapted and the results were documented in a book published in German.[1]

The book includes two parts: Part 1 compiles information and guidelines for the interaction with people affected by depression. Information is provided on the character of the disease depression, on factors leading to depression, and various therapeutic approaches that are available. A review of today's research on spirituality and depression describes how spiritual factors can impact depression positively and but also negatively. Chapters on conversation skills and pastoral counselling provide help for the interaction with people affected by depression. Part 2 offers information for planning of a thematic Sunday service including a sermon on theological aspects of depression; a Bible study on depression tackling questions like, "Does faith help to prevent depression? Is there a link between depression and guilt?"; suggestions for confirmation classes focusing on questions like, "What builds me up –what drags me down?"; a section proposing answers to "frequently asked questions."[2]

4 Participatory Implementation in Congregations

At the beginning of the project, the congregations in a church district in southern Germany were informed about the intended project and were invited to participate. Four of them expressed interest and asked for more details. In these congregations, members of the project team introduced the background and the planned implementation of the project to the respective parish councils. After

1 Birgit Weyel and Beate Jakob, eds., *Menschen mit Depressionen. Orientierungen und Impulse für die Praxis in Kirchengemeinden* (Gütersloh: Gütersloher Verlagshaus, 2014).
2 Cf. Weyel and Jakob, *Menschen mit Depressionen.*

this, three congregations confirmed their participation while one parish council withdrew. They found depression to be a very sensitive topic and felt that such a project would bear unpredictable risks and might completely overwhelm the congregation. In the congregations that finally committed themselves to the project, a participatory approach was applied. Each congregation formed a project group that was briefed about the background of the project and got some basic information about the nature of depression. The project group then invited representatives of the congregation (like pastors and volunteers leading groups of the congregation), health professionals from the diaconical services, general practitioners and pharmacists, and representatives of the civil society to a second meeting.

This group was invited to perform a mapping exercise. The participants created a map of the congregation and of secular groups/organizations within the congregation by identifying groups, important persons, meeting points that might play a role in tackling mental health issues, and noting them on cards. Different colors were chosen for church groups and secular entities. In addition, relationships between the various groups were marked by connecting the respective cards with lines.

The map they created showed the assets of the congregation and their links to other church or secular assets. Within the congregation they mapped, for example, women's groups, communication teams, grief groups, toddler groups, the kindergarten, a pastoral counselling team, etc. Among the secular entities that were put on the map were the general practitioner's surgery, the pharmacy, groups visiting terminally ill persons, etc. The lines marking the linkages between the assets showed that a good number of church groups were not well linked but worked in isolation.

This exercise was an eye-opener both for the congregation members and the representatives of the formal health system. Even the congregation members had not known all of the church activities and groups. Referring to a counselling group in the congregation a general practitioner said: "For some of my patients it is equally important to receive a contact address as to get a prescription. Now I know where to connect them." A pharmacist said: "So far, I have been aware of only about 20 percent of the groups existing here."

Already this first step of the project implementation had an important outcome: The congregations entered into a process of becoming aware of their assets to improve health, and of networking and establishing links to the formal health sector. One congregation meeting was attended by the promoter of an initiative of the civil community named "Healthy Community Eningen".[3] Here,

3 Eningen is a community in southern Germany.

important links to the civil society could be established during the very first meeting of the project group.

As a next step, the congregations were provided with information on the expectations of people affected by depression, based on initial project research.[4] The following information was shared:

- People suffering from depression suggest to provide sound information on the disease character of depression as they are tired of hearing sentences like, "Pull yourself together"; "It is a matter of will to overcome an episode of depression."
- They long for social support in a community where they feel safe.
- As many sick persons are not employed, they would appreciate opportunities to be active in the congregation. They wish to be included in activities having to take responsibility and to be expected to appear every day at a certain time.

Based on the mapping exercise and having the expectations of people with depression in mind, the project groups drafted an implementation plan for their particular congregations. The leading question was, "How can we meet the expectations of people with depression and their relatives within our congregation by using our own assets?"

Each of the implementation plans the congregations developed had a slightly different focus. One of the congregations chose the motto of "How can we promote healing accompaniment in our congregation?" Another one focused on the issue of "Depression and personal guilt". The project repeatedly initiated lively discussions among the congregation members who started to talk about depression and about how they could include persons they knew were suffering from depression. People said: "We have to be aware of who is missing in our services or in group meetings. Let's follow up on them instead of just leaving them aside because we feel unable to meet the expectations of a person who is deeply depressed."

Here are the main activities that were planned and implemented in the participating congregations:

- All congregations celebrated thematic Sunday services. These services provided an important platform to create awareness about the disease character of depression and the frequency of mental disorders so that people become aware that "Christians get depression, too," and that people affected by depression need professional therapy.

4 Cf. chapter II.3 in this volume: Beate Jakob, *Is Faith a Source of Strength? Do Congregations Offer Support? A Qualitative Study with People Affected by Mental Disorders and their Relatives.*

- In the congregations, health professionals offered lectures on depression in general, depression affecting the elderly, and depression and spirituality. These meetings provided information on the factors causing depression, the available treatment and the ways congregations can assist people affected by depression.
- Special offers for smaller groups included an art-therapy seminar and a seminar for relatives on "If the person next to me is depressed."
- Volunteers, such as group leaders and the members of an already existing counselling group were offered further trainings providing information about the nature of depression and mental disorders. Moreover they were taught conversation skills and pastoral counselling approaches.
- Confirmation classes about mobbing and depression were held.
- Biblical reflections on "depression and guilt," and on "depression as a biblical topic" were shared.
- In one of the congregations, the two pastors started offering informal counselling hours once a week and offered personal blessings after the Sunday service.
- After events or lectures, the participants shared personal issues in small groups ("safe spaces") instead of discussing the presented issues on an intellectual level in the large group.

In these congregations, issues of mental health were prominent during the project period lasting from six months up to one year. All offers were well received and the participants also included people who so far had not taken part in the life of the congregation or were not members. There was a very good media response. The local newspapers and some radio stations and television stations invited members of the project team and of the participating congregations for interviews.

5 Reflections and Recommendations

In reflective meetings following the project time, the pastors and congregation members articulated their high appreciation of the project. Asked about the benefits of the project, many congregation members mentioned the access to information about the disease, its various causes, the impact on people's lives and available therapies. Thus, awareness was created about the frequency of depression among congregation members, and misconceptions in congregations concerning mental disorders were addressed. One person mentioned: "It's been good to openly address issues around depression. It had been a taboo in spite of all of us knowing depression being a major problem within the congregation. We even have started to openly talk about suicide." A 40 year old women suffering from depression very much appreciated that instead of just promoting praying for people suffering from depression, the project had focused on sensitizing and informing. Therefore, she dared to openly talk about her experiences and through this, she no longer felt stigmatized by the congregation.

All pastors admitted that they had not expected people suffering from depression and their relatives to disclose so much and to actively take part in such a project instead of congregation members only discussing about depression on an intellectual level. They also mentioned that the project helped them to become sensitive for signs and symptoms of depression and to become aware of the frequency of depression among congregation members. Therefore, depression had become a major issue in their practice of pastoral counselling.

Giving a summary, one of the pastors said: "Definitely, a congregation has health promoting assets. We should not underestimate them. Among these assets are social support, safe spaces, and rituals like personal blessings. Especially the two latter are specific for religious communities and can't be offered by secular communities. We have the capacity to accompany and support people with mental disorders, sometimes by just listening to them and making them aware that 'We see you and we understand your pain.' Others we can assist by referring them to health professionals. Of course, we need to be humble and sometimes it's been like getting into a dead end. But we have embarked on a journey towards assisting sick congregation members by using our own assets."

Some activities continued after the project phase came to an end. For example, in one congregation people received further training in counselling. Another one still offers a safe space for people seeking advice and counselling once a month after the Sunday service. Thus, a process of transformation started whereby people with depression or other mental health disorders and their relatives feel at home in a congregation that offers a safe space for them.

Representatives of the local "Alliance against Depression" were very impressed by congregations taking up the issue. They regard the project as the starting point of a fruitful cooperation between the congregations and the formal health sector.

Based on the experiences with the pilot projects, other German congregations are getting involved in a similar project. Widening the thematic area of the project, six German congregations have committed themselves to search for ways of "Promoting Mental Health in our Congregation."

Vandana Kanth

"Nayi Roshni" – "New Light" for People Suffering from Mental Disorders

A Community-Based Mental Health Care Project in Raxaul, Bihar, India

In 2014, the Duncan Hospital in Raxaul, India, started the mental health project "Nayi Roshni" ("New Light" in Hindi) to address the growing rate of suicides in the area. Until 2014, the hospital had not offered any mental health services.

The Christian Duncan Hospital evolved from a small clinic founded by the Scottish medical missionary Dr. Cecil Duncan in 1930. Over time it developed into a 200 bed hospital that today provides quality health care to the people of northern Bihar and neighbouring Nepal. Duncan Hospital belongs to the Emmanuel Hospital Association which is a fellowship of Christian institutions and individuals with the mission to transform communities through caring, with a primary emphasis on the poor and the marginalized.

In the early 1990s, the hospital started the Community Health and Development Programme. With its integrated approach towards health and development, this programme responds to the health needs of communities like nutrition, HIV and AIDS, disabilities, mother and child health, anti-trafficking initiatives, noncommunicable diseases. Since 2014, through the Nayi Roshni Project, the programme responds to mental health issues.

1 Raxaul – A Difficult Place to Live

Raxaul is a town in the East Champaran District of the Indian state of Bihar close to the border of Nepal. This district is characterized by high rates of unemployment, illiteracy and landlessness. It contains a major transport route that runs between Kathmandu and Calcutta.

Because of the lack of land, industries and job opportunities most of the common men are daily wage workers (which depends on availability of work in the area) or have small shops where they sell tea, pan or other commodities. Though Bihar state government has declared the state as 'Dry state' with the prohibition of sale and consumption of alcohol, being a border area alcohol consumption is seen in many pockets. Drug usage and prostitution in the border areas have led to a fairly high prevalence of HIV and AIDS.

https://doi.org/10.1515/9783110674217-012

The social status of women and young girls is very low. Women are expected to do all the household work. Many of them are illiterate and have very little decision-making power. Their health status deteriorates with long working hours, poor diet and frequent pregnancies. Children, especially boys are mostly considered to be a source of income, and it is easy to find child laborers in many shops & hotels.

2 Why the Mental Health Project at Duncan Hospital Was Started

2.1 Mental Health in India and in Bihar

According to data of the National Mental Health Programme (NMHP) in India, 6.5 per cent of the population suffers from acute or chronic mental disorders which equals nearly 70 million people.[1] The main psychiatric sufferings in the adult population consist of acute, chronic or frequently recurring mental disorders, emotional disorders such as anxiety, hysteria, neurotic depression, alcohol abuse, alcohol and drug dependence; psychiatric disorders among children are also present. Most of these patients live in rural areas, far away from any mental health facility.

In the society, there are still many misconceptions related to mental diseases. Among these are:

- Mental deseases are caused through the "bad eye" of jealous neighbours or people who performed a ritual which has attracted bad spirits to enter a particular person. Symptoms of mental diseases are related to the behavior of a bad spirit in a person.
- Mentally ill patients are dangerous and prone to crime.
- Mental disease is a punishment because he or she has committed some wrong either in this life or in the past.
- People with mental diseases will never get better. Therefore, it does not make a difference if they get treatment or not.

These misconceptions lead to stigmatization and discrimination of people affected by mental disorders in the Indian society. As some mentally ill persons

1 Suman K. Sinha and Jagdish Kaur, "National mental health programme: Manpower development scheme of eleventh five-year plan," *Indian J Psychiatry* (2011 Jul–Sep; 53[3]): 261–265, in URL: https://www.ncbi.nlm.nih.gov/pmc/articles/PMC3221186/ (last accessed on 1 April 2020).

cannot care for themselves, their families sometimes regard them as a burden or curse. Often, families hide mentally ill family members and do not dare to talk about the disease. Many mentally ill people are seen bound in chains.

2.2 The Mental Health Treatment Gap

According to WHO,[2] the number of people with psychosis, bipolar disorders, and moderate to severe depression who have access to treatment in lower middle-income countries is about 10 times lower than the corresponding number of patients in high-income countries.

Despite this apparent treatment gap, most African and Southeast Asian countries, on the average, spend only about 1 USD per capita for mental health – compared to more than 80 USD per capita in high income countries.[3] Many developing countries still struggle with the consequences of infectious diseases, malnutrition and infant and maternal mortality and hence, mental health is given low priority in the competition for scarce health resources.

Still, there are additional factors that deter people from seeking care for mental disorders in developing countries. For example, poor knowledge and stigma within the community often prevent people with mental disorders or epilepsy and their families from seeking help.[4]

India with a population of over a billion people has a staggering number of only 3.500 psychiatrists. The entire mental health workforce, comprising clinical psychiatrists, psychologists, psychiatric social workers and psychiatric nurses stands at 7.000, while the actual requirement is 54.750.[5] That means there is only one psychiatrist for more than 340.000 people. As most of these work in urban settings, professionals are even less present in rural communities. Up to 2014, no psychiatrist was available in Raxaul.

Lack of psychiatrists and other adequate mental health services plus the above mentioned misconceptions are the reasons why the primary contacts for people with mental diseases in rural areas are generally traditional and/or faith-healers.

---

2 WHO, "Mental Health Atlas 2017," *World Health Organization* (2018): 45.

3 WHO, "Mental Health Atlas 2017," 27.

4 Cf. Oye Gureje, Victor O. Lasebikan VO, Olusola Ephraim-Oluwanuga, Benjamin O. Olley and Lola Kola, "Community study of knowledge of and attitude to mental illness in Nigeria," *The British Journal of Psychiatry 186* (2005 May; 186): 436–441.

5 Cf. Janani Sampath, "TNN," *The Times of India* (Jan 20, 2014).

2.3 Increasing Trend of Suicides

Globally, suicide is one of the leading causes of death, especially in the age group of 15–35 years. Nearly 60 per cent of these deaths are among young adults in their productive years of life.[6]

In India, in the last two decades the suicide rate has increased from 7.9 to 10.3 per 100.000 per year, with varying rates across the country. The southern states of Kerala, Karnataka, Andhra Pradesh and Tamil Nadu have a suicide rate of more than 15, while in the northern states of Punjab, Uttar Pradesh, Bihar, Jammu and Kashmir, the rate is less than 3. Each year more than 100.000 lives are lost to suicide.[7]

A study from the South East Asian Region of WHO reported that individuals who have a slightly higher risk for attempting suicide may not necessarily have a serious mental disorder, but include those who are unemployed, who are victims of domestic violence, have conflicts within themselves or with other family members on a continual basis and those recently discharged from hospitals. The latter group comprises people with mental disorders but also terminal illnesses such as cancer, HIV and AIDS, and Tuberculosis.[8]

There is little data available about the rate of suicides in Bihar and the motives behind these attempts. To gain a better perspective on this issue, over the past year Duncan Hospital has been collecting data on the number of suicide attempts that were admitted to the hospital. An unpublished study was conducted in 2010 where the information from 2007–2009 was studied. Figure 1 describes the trend over the years.

Another unpublished study showed: From February 2011 to January 2012, 418 attempted suicides were committed accounting for about 9.5 per cent of adult medical inpatient workload – again a huge increase in numbers compared to the data of 2007 to 2009. 35 per cent of these inpatients were admitted to the intensive care unit where costs for advanced life support are extremely high for individuals and their families.[9] The suicide rates between males and females

6 SEARO – WHO, *Suicide Prevention: Emerging from Darkness* (2001), in URL: http://apps.searo.who.int/PDS_DOCS/B0754.pdf (last accessed on 1 April 2020).

7 Cf. Lakshmi Vijaykumar, "Suicide and its prevention: the urgent need in India," *Indian J Psychiatry 49* (2007): 81–84.

8 SEARO – WHO, *Suicide Prevention: Emerging from Darkness* (2001), in URL: http://apps.searo.who.int/PDS_DOCS/B0754.pdf (last accessed on 1 April 2020).

9 In private facilities in India, patients usually have to pay for the treatment costs out of their own pocket.

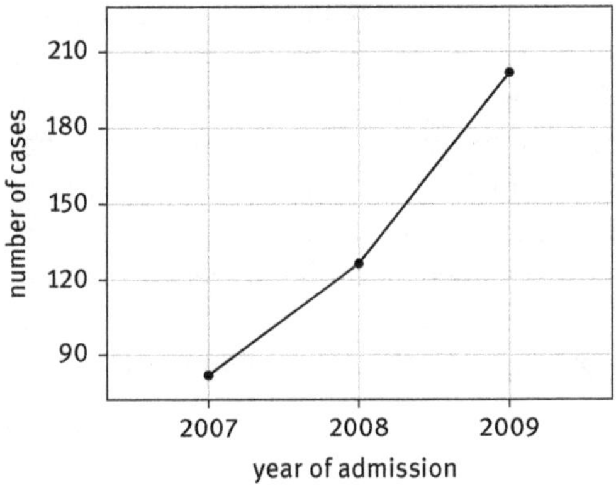

Figure 1: Number of patients after suicide attempts admitted to Duncan Hospital, 2007–2009 (unpublished).

were approximately equal at 47.9 per cent and 52.1 per cent respectively. Perhaps because of the medical-legal issues involved in reporting suicides to the authorities, most of the patients seen were from Nepal (82.6 per cent) and only 17.4 per cent were from India.

Extended interviews were carried out with 157 survivors of suicide and one or two of their relatives. 80 per cent of the survivors were below the age of 30. In the interviews, it was found that the major reasons for suicide were familial conflicts (more than 80 per cent). 18 per cent were found to have depression[10] and 4 per cent had an underlying serious mental disorder like schizophrenia and psychosis (unpublished study).

2.4 Domestic Violence and High Prevalence of Alcoholism

Domestic violence is a fact of life in all societies and across all cultures, irrespective of economic status and education. Bihar is the state in India with the highest prevalence of domestic violence and alcohol abuse. A survey on domestic violence[11] showed a high incidence and prevalence of domestic abuse and

10 This study used the ICD (International Classification of Diseases) 10 depression inventory to identify the depression rate among the respondents.
11 Cf. Vandana Kanth, *Duncan Hospital, Community Health and Development Programme, Needs assessment on domestic violence in Raxaul Block* (unpublished study, 2011).

violence in Raxaul Block.[12] There is also a high linkage between alcohol usage and domestic violence.

WHO data[13] show that victims of domestic violence are two times as likely to experience depression, 16 per cent more likely to have low birth-weight babies, 1.5 times more prone to be infected with HIV. 38 percent of all murders of women were reported as being committed by a male intimate partner.

There is strong evidence that a large component of the higher rates of depression and anxiety found among women is connected to their lower social value and reduced decision-making power in families and communities.

3 Nayi Roshni – A Pilot Project to Break the Silence and to Benefit People with Mental Disorders and Their Relatives

In 2014 the Duncan Hospital launched the Nayi Roshni project as part of its Community Health and Development Programme. This project is the first of its kind in the catchment area of Duncan Hospital.

The goal of this community-based project is to improve the situation of people suffering from mental disorders in the Raxaul area by working with and in communities. The project has three objectives:

- To empower communities to understand mental health and its social determinants (like alcoholism, domestic violence, debt, gender issues etc.).
- To reduce the stigma associated with mental disorders.
- To improve access to mental health services in the area.

3.1 Formation of a Project Team and of Task Force Groups

The project started with the selection of appropriate project staff who were motivated enough and had a heart to work on mental health and its social

12 According to the administrative structure in India, a block is a sub-division of a district (which is a sub-division of a state). It comprises a number of villages.

13 Cf. WHO fact sheets on mental health (updated March 2018), in URL: https://www.who.int/news-room/fact-sheets/detail/mental-health-strengthening-our-response (last accessed on 1 April 2020).

determinants. These persons received a training as even among health professionals, knowledge about diagnosis and treatment of mental disorders is low. A mental health nurse from New Zealand trained six project staff who learnt how to diagnose and treat common mental disorders and how to mobilize communities. These trained staff members have formed a project team to steer the project.

Nayi Roshni implements various interventions to sensitize and teach individuals, communities and organizations towards understanding the social determinants of mental health and various mental disorders. The project team promotes sensitization among families, groups (women's groups, girls' and boys' groups), caregivers of people with mental disorders, government primary health workers, religious leaders, community leaders, etc. In addition, mass sensitization is done through rallies, skits, dramas and role plays during the celebration of mental health days, which includes World Suicide Prevention Day.

Project team members formed self-help groups of people with mental disorders and their caregivers that they accompany.

As a main characteristic of Nayi Roshni, local people work with and for their own people. So-called Task Forces form the backbone of the project. Each of the participating communities builds up a Task Force consisting of four men and four women who are chosen by the communities themselves. To date, 65 Task Force Groups comprising about 520 members are active in the communities.

The Task Force members receive training about mental health and its social determinants. This training enables them to teach groups and to interact with people suffering from mental disorders. The Task Forces sensitize their communities and create awareness about mental health through rallies, videos, and role plays. As the Task Force members live in the communities, they can identify people suffering from mental disorders or being at risk of developing a mental disorder in their day-to-day interactions or through home visits. The Task Force Groups address local issues related to domestic violence, familial conflicts, alcoholism and suicidal attempts. They can help to deal with issues about the rights of people living with mental disorders. Moreover, they identify and refer patients to the hospital for adequate management.

The Task Forces have identified many patients in need of treatment for a mental health issue, but they also saw that the majority of them did not have the money for medical treatment. In response, members of the Roshni project team led a discussion in the Task Force Groups about how they could help poor people. Ten Task Force Group members became motivated to address the problem and decided that they would begin saving some money that could be used for people who are poor. The Roshni Project gave them a small metal box with a lock and key and the groups started contributing money. In addition, they have also started motivating other community members to put money into the savings box. In the evenings, when people of the village are sitting and talking outside, members of the Task Force Groups circulate around the village and invite people to make a contribution. In this way, they are collecting funds that can be used to help needy members of their own community.

The Task Forces form a link between the communities and the hospital. On a monthly basis, the Nayi Roshni project team meets with them to hear about people who are at risk of developing a mental disorder in their communities. The project group conducts home visits to these people and assesses the situation of the person and his or her family. Members of the project group also do follow-ups of people with mental disorders in the communities.

After its first year of implementation, the project has encouraged the hospital to recruit a psychiatrist who was the first and only psychiatrist in the whole of East Champaran District. The hospital has established a mental health unit and now is able to meet the increased demand for mental health services created by the activities at community level. Currently, the Nayi Roshni Project consists of nine staff, which includes a clinical psychologist and a driver. The clinical psychologist was hired as part of a response to the growing need of field level counsellings, drop-out patients and for those not willing to avail mental health services at the base hospital.

3.2 Whole Person Care

Duncan Hospital is driven by the motto of "Whole Person Care" as we believe that a person consists of body, soul, and spirit that form a unity. Therefore, to cater to one's need holistically it is important to look at the whole person with all his or her relationships. In addition to providing treatment for the body, it is also important to take care of his or her emotional and spiritual health. All patients who are involved in our mental health project receive both emotional and spiritual counselling which lifts them up and helps them to recover. Most of the time such, counselling is done in the presence of the members of the patients' families and or other relatives which helps not only the patients but also those who are related to them.

To improve the economic situation of people with mental disorders the project activities include an income generating programme for them. They are also assisted when they apply for government entitlements.

3.3 Nayi Roshni Changes People's Lives

The following examples show how Nayi Roshni brings light to the lives of individuals and their families.[14]

In Raghauta village a widow struggles to raise her six children. Priyanka, her 14-year-old daughter, who was having some problems in her life, suddenly made a decision to take poison. When the village Task Force Group became aware of the situation, they hired a vehicle to bring the girl to Duncan Hospital. For several days, she struggled for her life in the intensive care unit. Members of the Task Force Group came regularly to encourage the mother who sat waiting for her daughter to recover. After eleven days, the family was asked to pay the hospital bill of Rs. 26.000. The mother sold her jewellery and sought help from people in her community and in this way was able to pay the bill. Though the girl was still quite sick and needed continued intensive care, the mother wanted to take her home because she had exhausted her financial resources. In this situation, the Task Force Group together with a member of the Roshni staff urged the mother to keep the patient in the hospital and promised to help her. After five more days the girl had improved so much that she was now ready to go home. The hospital bill amounted to a further Rs. 27.000. Seeing the need, one of the Task Force Group members took an interest-free loan from the village women's self-help group and gave it to the mother to pay the hospital bill. The hospital gave a Rs. 5.000 donation so that the bill could be paid. Today, the daughter is doing very well.

Another example is the story of Shrimati: She has a daughter and two sons, one of whom is married. The entire family lives together including her married son and daughter-in-law. Kundan, her husband, is a day-labourer and has been a heavy drinker for many years. Most days, after work, he drank excessively, and then returned home. Once at home, he shouted at Shrimati and the children and often beat them. Shrimati thought that when her children were older, his behavior would improve, but this was not the case. Over time, she lost hope. She planned to commit suicide by poisoning herself, and she started to secretly store some poison at home until one day she took the poison. One of the Task Force Group members of New Roshni project lives next door and when she heard what Shrimati had done, she came to her house and urged the family to take her to Duncan Hospital. So fortunately her life was saved. Back at home she shared her experiences with the other Task Force Group members who encouraged her and counselled her against suicide. Her husband was shocked when he realized the desperate situation of his wife that had led her to attempt suicide. He was open

14 All names mentioned in the case stories have been changed.

enough to talk to the Task Force Group members and over time reduced his drinking. It also helped that at the same time the government passed a law prohibiting alcohol in Bihar so that alcoholism was discussed among the people. Today, Kundan's behavior at home is much better and he is very friendly with other community members. The family's economic situation improved as Kundan now spends much less money on alcohol. His example also helped other men to reduce their drinking.

These examples show how the Nayi Roshni project changes the lives of individuals and families. The silence around mental health has been broken, stigma and discrimination are being addressed and access to mental health services is about to be improved.

It is our hope that this project will provide a role model for community-based mental health care in rural India that will then be implemented in other blocks of East Champaran.

Contributors

Dr. Annette Haußmann is a junior professor for Practical Theology with focus on Pastoral Care in Heidelberg (Ruprecht-Karls-University) and psychological psychotherapist for cognitive behavioral therapy (in training).

Dr. Beate Jakob is consultant for health and healing at the German Institute for Medical Mission (DIFÄM) in Tuebingen.

Dr. Vandana Kanth is a medical doctor and works as Director of the Department for Community Health & Development Projects of the Duncan Hospital in East Champaran District of Bihar, India.

Dr. Constantin Klein is a professor for Spiritual Care at the Clinic and Policlinic for Palliative Medicine at Ludwig Maximilians University Munich.

Dr. Michael Klessmann is a professor emeritus for Practical Theology at the Theological Seminary Wuppertal/Bethel.

Paul Mekani is principal nursing officer at the Nkhoma Hospital, Lilongwe District, Malawi.

Japhet Myaba is holder of a Master of Public Health and works as a Mental Health Project Coordinator at Malawi Council for the Handicapped.

Dr. Birgit Weyel is a professor for Practical Theology with focus on Pastoral Care and Pastoral Theology at the Faculty of Protestant Theology in Tuebingen (Eberhard Karls University).

Dr. Dr. Christian Zwingmann is a professor for Empirical Social Research at the Protestant University of Applied Sciences in Bochum.

https://doi.org/10.1515/9783110674217-013

Bibliography

Abdallah, Mahmoud. “Religion, Gesellschaft und Moralwerte: Umma zwischen Heterogenität der Gegenwart und dem Traum von Einheit.” *Ökumenische Rundschau* 65 (2016): 213–226.

Alavi, Seyedeh Z., Forogh Amin and Azar P. Savoji. “Relationship between Pathological Guilt and God Image with Depression in Cancer Patients.” *Procedia – Social and Behavioral Sciences* 84 (2013): 919–924.

Albertsen, Elizabeth J., Lynn E. O’Connor and Jack W. Berry. “Religion and interpersonal guilt: Variations across ethnicity and spirituality.” *Mental Health, Religion and Culture* 9(1) (2006): 67–84.

Alem, Atalay, Lars Jacobsson and Charlotte Hanlon. “Community-based mental health care in Africa: mental health workers’ views.” *Journal of World Psychiatry* 7(1) (2008): 54.

Alem, Atalay. “Community-based vs. hospital-based mental health care: the case of Africa.” *World Psychiatry* 1(2) (2002): 98–99.

Allport, Gordon W. and J. Michael Ross. “Personal religious orientation and prejudice.” *Journal of Personality and Social Psychology* 5 (1967): 432–443.

Allwinn, Sabine. “Krankheitsbewältigung als individueller, interaktiver und sozialer Prozess.” In *Psychosoziale Dienste und Seelsorge im Krankenhaus*, edited by Christoph Schneider-Harpprecht and Sabine Allwinn, 17–104. Göttingen: Vandenhoeck & Ruprecht, 2005.

Andersson, Gerhard. “Chronic pain and praying to a higher power. Useful or useless?” *Journal of Religion and Health* 47 (2008): 176–187.

Ando, Michiyo, Tatsuya Morita, Tatsuo Akechi and Takuya Okamoto. “Efficacy of short-term life-review interviews on the spiritual well-being of terminal ill cancer patients.” *Journal of Pain and Symptom Management* 39 (2010): 993–1002.

Angst, Jules, Alex Gamma, M. Gastpar, Jean-Pierre Lépine, J. Mendlewicz and A. Tylee. “Gender differences in depression. Epidemiological findings from the European DEPRES I and II studies.” *European Archives of Psychiatry and Clinical Neuroscience* 252(5) (2002): 201–209.

Ano, Gene G. and Erin B. Vasconcelles. “Religious coping and psychosocial adjustment to stress: A meta-analysis.” *Journal of Clinical Psychology* 61 (2005): 1–20.

Antonovsky, Aaron. “The structure and properties of the Sense of Coherence Scale.” *Social Science & Medicine* 36 (1993): 725–733.

Antonovsky, Aaron. *Health, Stress and Coping*. San Francisco: Jossey-Bass, 1979.

Asser, Seth M. and Rita Swan. “Child fatalities from religion-motivated medical neglect.” *Pediatrics* 101 (1998): 625–629.

Bade, Jörg. *Depression und Segen. Zur seelsorgerlichen Begegnung mit depressiven Menschen*. Münster: Lit Verlag, 2000.

Barnard, Laura K. and John F. Curry. “The Relationship of Clergy Burnout to Self-Compassion and Other Personality Dimensions.” *Pastoral Psychology* 61(2) (2012): 149–163.

Barton, Yakov A., Lisa Miller, Priya Wickramaratne, Marc J. Gameroff and Myrna M. Weissman. “Religious attendance and social adjustment as protective against depression: A 10-year prospective study.” *Journal of Affective Disorders* 146(1) (2013): 53–57.

Batson, C. Daniel, Patricia Schoenrade and W. Larry Ventis. *Religion and the individual. A social-psychological perspective*. New York: Oxford University Press, 1993.

https://doi.org/10.1515/9783110674217-014

Bäumer, Regina and Michael Plattig, eds. *Dunkle Nacht und Depression*. Ostfildern: Grünewald, 2008.

Bay, Paul S., Daniel Beckman, James Trippi, Richard Gunderman and Colin Terry. “The effect of pastoral care services on anxiety, depression, hope, religious coping, and religious problem solving styles: a randomized controlled study.” *Journal of Religion and Health* 47(1) (2008): 57–69.

Beck, Aaron T. *Cognitive therapy of depression*. Chichester: Wiley, 1979.

Benson, Herbert. *Heilung durch Glauben*. München: Heyne, 1997.

Benson, Peter L. “Religion and substance use.” In *Religion and mental health*, edited by John F. Schumaker, 211–220. New York: Oxford University Press, 1992.

Berger, Klaus. “Biblisches Christentum als Heilungsreligion.” In *Heilung – Energie – Geist. Heilung zwischen Wissenschaft, Religion und Geschäft*, edited by Werner Heinz Ritter and Bernhard Wolf, 226–246. Göttingen: Vandenhoeck & Ruprecht, 2005.

Bertelsmann Stiftung, ed. *Religionsmonitor 2008*. Gütersloh: Bertelsmann Stiftung, 2009.

Bjørkløf, Guro H., Knut Engedal, Geir Selbæk, Siren E. Kouwenhoven and Anne-Sofie Helvik. “Coping and depression in old age: A literature review.” *Dementia and Geriatric Cognitive Disorders* 35 (2013): 121–154.

Boettcher, Birthe. “Spiritual Care und die multiprofessionelle Zusammenarbeit von Seelsorgern und Psychotherapeuten im ambulanten Kontext.” *Spiritual Care* 7 (2018): 377–385.

Bonelli, Raphael M. “Suizid und Religiosität.” In *Psychotherapie und Spiritualität: Mit existenziellen Konflikten und Transzendenzfragen professionell umgehen*, edited by Michael Utsch, Raphael M. Bonelli and Samuel Pfeifer, 133–142. Berlin/Heidelberg: Springer, 2014.

Bonelli, Raphael and Harold G. Koenig. “Mental disorders, religion and spirituality 1990 to 2010: A systematic evidence-based review.” *Journal of Religion and Health* 52 (2013): 657–673.

Borman, Patricia L. and David N. Dixon. “Spirituality and the 12 steps of substance abuse recovery.” *Journal of Psychology and Theology* 26 (1998): 287–291.

Bowie, Cameron. “The burden of diseases in Malawi.” *Malawi Medical Journal* 18(3) (2006): 103–110.

Braam, Aarjan W. “Religion und Depression.” In *Gesundheit – Religion – Spiritualität*, edited by Constantin Klein, Hendrik Berth and Friedrich Balck, 273–290. Weinheim: Beltz Juventa, 2011.

Braam, Aarjan W., Aartjan T. Beekman and Pieter van den Eeden et al. “Religious climate and geographical distribution of depressive symptoms in older Dutch citizens.” *Journal of Affective Disorders* 54(1–2) (1999): 149–159.

Braam, Aarjan W., Dorly J. Deeg, Jan L. Poppelaars, Aartjan T. Beekman and Willem van Tilburg. “Prayer and depressive symptoms in a period of secularization: patterns among older adults in the Netherlands.” *American Journal of Geriatric Psychiatry* 15 (2007): 273–281.

Braam, Aarjan W., E. Hein, Dorly J. H. Deeg, J. W. R. Twisk, Aartjan T. Beekman and Willem van Tilburg. “Religious Involvement and 6-Year Course of Depressive Symptoms in Older Dutch Citizens: Results from the Longitudinal Aging Study Amsterdam.” *Journal of Aging and Health* 16(4) (2004): 467–489.

Braam, Aarjan W., Martin J. Prince and Aartjan T. Beekman et al. “Physical health and depressive symptoms in older Europeans. Results from EURODEP.” *The British Journal of Psychiatry* 187 (2005): 35–42.

Braam, Aarjan W., Hanneke Schaap-Jonker and Marleen H. L. van der Horst et al. “Twelve-year history of late-life depression and subsequent feelings to God.” *The American Journal of Geriatric Psychiatry* 22(11) (2014): 1272–1281.

Brakemeier, Eva-Lotta, Claus Normann and Mathias Berger. “Ätiopathogenese der unipolaren Depression.” Bundesgesundheitsblatt-Gesundheitsforschung-Gesundheitsschutz 51(4) (2008): 379–391.

Bucher, Anton. *Die dunkle Seite der Kirche*. Etsdorf: Galia, 2010.

Bucher, Anton A. “Zornig und strafend – oder zu milde? Negative Gottesbilder.” In *Religiosität: Die dunkle Seite: Beiträge zur empirischen Religionsforschung*, edited by Christian Zwingmann, Constantin Klein and Florian Jeserich, 23–42. Münster/New York: Waxmann, 2017.

Buggle, Franz. “Warum gibt es (fast) keine deutsche empirische Religionspsychologie?” *Forschungsberichte des Psychologischen Instituts der Albert-Ludwigs-Universität Freiburg i. Br. 73* (1991).

Büssing, Arndt. “Empirische Zugänge zum Beten.” In *Gebet als Resonanzereignis. Annäherungen im Horizont von Spiritual Care*, edited by Simon Peng-Keller, 111–128. Göttingen: Vandenhoeck & Ruprecht, 2017.

Büssing, Arndt, Federico Baiocco and Klaus Baumann. “Spiritual Dryness in Catholic Laypersons Working as Volunteers is Related to Reduced Life Satisfaction Rather than to Indicators of Spirituality.” *Pastoral Psychology* 67(1) (2018): 1–15.

Büssing, Arndt, Jochen Sautermeister, Eckhard Frick and Klaus Baumann. “Reactions and Strategies of German Catholic Priests to Cope with Phases of Spiritual Dryness.” *Journal of Religion and Health* 56 (2017): 1018–1031.

Butler, Lisa D., Lynn C. Waelde, Andrew D. Hastings, Xin-Hua Chen, Barbara Symons et al. “Meditation with yoga, group therapy with hypnosis, and psychoeducation for long-term depressed mood: A randomized pilot trial.” *Journal of Clinical Psychology* 64 (2008): 806–820.

Chatters, Linda M., Kai M. Bullard, Robert J. Taylor and Amanda T. Woodward et al. “Religious participation and DSM-IV disorders among older African Americans: Findings from the National Survey of American Life.” *The American Journal of Geriatric Psychiatry* 16(12) (2008): 957–965.

Chatters, Linda M., Robert J. Taylor, Amanda T. Woodward and Emily J. Nicklett. “Social support from church and family members and depressive symptoms among older African Americans.” *The American Journal of Geriatric Psychiatry* 23(6) (2015): 559–567.

Chida, Yoishi, Andrew Steptoe and Lynda H. Powell. “Religiosity/spirituality and mortality.” *Psychotherapy and Psychosomatics* 78 (2009): 81–90.

Cochrane, Jim. “Religious Health Assets (RHAs) – Conceptual and Theoretical Framework.” In *Religion, Faith and Public Health. Documentation on a Consultation held at Difäm*, edited by Difäm, German Institute for Medical Mission, 14–45. Tübingen, 9–11 February 2006.

Colucci, Erminia and Graham Martin. “Religion and spirituality along the suicidal path.” *Suicide Life Threat Behavior* 38 (2008): 229–244.

Coppinger Pickett, Candace, Justin L. Barrett, Cynthia B. Eriksson and Christina Kabiri. “Social Networks among Ministry Relationships: Relational Capacity, Burnout, & Ministry Effectiveness.” *Journal of Psychology and Theology* 45(2) (2017): 92–105.

Corrigan, Patrick W. and Amy C. Watson. “Understanding the impact of stigma on people with mental illness.” *World Psychiatry* 1(1) (2002): 16–20.

Cotton, Sian, Daniel H. Grossoehme and Joel Tsevat. "Religion/spirituality and health in adolescents." In *Spirit, science and health. How the spiritual mind fuels physical wellness*, edited by Thomas G. Plante and Carl E. Thoresen, 143–156. Westport, CT: Praeger, 2007.

Culligan, Kevin. "Vom Umgang mit der Dunkelheit in der geistlichen Begleitung." In *'Dunkle Nacht' und Depression: Geistliche und psychische Krisen verstehen und unterscheiden*, edited by Regina Bäumer and Michael Plattig, 58–74. Ostfildern: Grünewald, 2008.

Curtis J. VanderWaal, Edwin I. Hernandez and Alix R. Sandman. "The gatekeepers: Involvement of Christian clergy in referrals and collaboration with Christian social workers and other helping professionals." *Social Work and Christianity* 39(1) (2012): 27–51.

De Lely, A. A., Walter W. van den Broek, Paul G. Mulder and Tom K. Birkenhäger. "Symptomen bij een depressie; bevindelijk gereformeerde versus niet-kerkelijke patiënten [Symptoms of depression in strict Calvinist patients and in patients without religious affiliations: a comparison]." *Tijdschrift voor psychiatrie* 51(5) (2009): 279–289.

Depping, Klaus. *Depressive alte Menschen seelsorgerlich begleiten. Auswege aus Schwermut und Verzweiflung*. Hannover: Lutherisches Verlagshaus, 2000.

Dervic, Kanita, Juan J. Carballo and Enrique Baca-Garcia et al. "Moral or religious objections to suicide may protect against suicidal behavior in bipolar disorder." *The Journal of Clinical Psychiatry* 72(10) (2011): 1390–1396.

Dervic, Kanita, Maria A. Oquendo and Michael F. Grunebaum et al. "Religious affiliation and suicide attempt." *American Journal of Psychiatry* 161 (2004): 2303–2308.

Donahue, Michael J. "Intrinsic and extrinsic religiousness: Review and meta-analysis." *Journal of Personality and Social Psychology* 48 (1985): 55–67.

Dörr, Anette. *Religiosität und Depression: Eine empirisch-psychologische Untersuchung*. Weinheim: Deutscher Studien-Verlag, 1987.

Dörr, Annette. *Religiosität und psychische Gesundheit. Zur Zusammenhangsstruktur spezifischer religiöser Konzepte*. Studienreihe psychologische Forschungsergebnisse 80. Hamburg: Verlag Dr. Kovač, 2001.

Dörr, Anette. "Religiöses Coping als Ressource bei der Bewältigung von Life Events." In *Religiosität: Messverfahren und Studien zu Gesundheit und Lebensbewältigung. Neue Beiträge zur Religionspsychologie*, edited by Christian Zwingmann and Helfried Moosbrugger, 261–276. Münster: Waxmann, 2004.

Drechsel, Wolfgang. *Gemeindeseelsorge*. Leipzig: Evangelische Verlagsanstalt, 2nd ed. 2016.

Due, Noel and Kirsten Due. "Courage and comfort for pastors in need." *Lutheran Theological Journal* 52(3) (2018): 128–140.

Dreyer, Yolanda. "Material poverty and the poverty of excess: Meaning-making as healing in an era of supermodernism." In *Pluralisation and social change. Dynamics of lived religion in South Africa and in Germany*. Praktische Theologie im Wissenschaftsdiskurs 21, edited by Lars Charbonnier, Johan Cilliers, Matthias Mader, Cas Wepener and Birgit Weyel, 75–87. Berlin: De Gruyter, 2018.

Ehm, Simone and Michael Utsch. "Glaube und Gesundheit. Historische Zusammenhänge und aktuelle Befunde." *EZW-Texte* 181 (2005): 5–16.

Ehrenberg, Alan. *Das erschöpfte Selbst: Depression und Gesellschaft in der Gegenwart*. Frankfurter Beiträge zur Soziologie und Sozialphilosophie 6. Frankfurt/Main: Campus, 2004.

EKD, ed. *Engagement und Indifferenz. Kirchenmitgliedschaft als soziale Praxis. V. EKD-Erhebung über Kirchenmitgliedschaft*. Hannover 2014.

Enright, Robert D. *Vergebung als Chance: Neuen Mut fürs Leben finden*. Bern: Hogrefe, 2006.
Ernst, Heiko. „Bindung und Lebensglück. Wie frühe Erfahrungen im Leben prägen.“ *Psychologie Heute* 32 (2005): 21–22.
Escher, Daniel. “How does religion promote forgiveness? Linking beliefs, orientations, and practices.” *Journal for the Scientific Study of Religion* 52(1) (2013): 100–119.
Exline, Julie J. “Belief in heaven and hell among Christians in the United States: Denominational differences and clinical implications.” *Journal of Death and Dying* 47(2) (2003): 155–168.
Exline, Julie J. “Religious and spiritual struggles.” In *APA handbook of psychology, religion, and spirituality*, edited by Kenneth I. Pargament et al., 459–475. Washington, DC: American Psychological Association, 2013.
Exline, Julie J., Kalman J. Kaplan and Joshua B. Grubbs. “Anger exit and assertion: Do people see protest toward God as morally acceptable?” *Psychology of Religion and Spirituality* 4(4) (2012): 264–277.
Exline, Julie J., Steven J. Krause and Karen A. Broer, “Spiritual Struggle Among Patients Seeking Treatment for Chronic Headaches: Anger and Protest Behaviors Toward God.” *Journal of Religion and Health* 55(5) (2016): 1729–1747.
Exline, Julie J., Kenneth I. Pargament., Joshua B. Grubbs and Anne Marie Yali. “The Religious and Spiritual Struggles Scale: Development and initial validation.” *Psychology of Religion and Spirituality* 6(3) (2014): 208–222.
Exline, Julie J., Crystal L. Park, Joshua M. Smyth and Michael P. Carey. “Anger toward God: Social-cognitive predictors, prevalence, and links with adjustment to bereavement and cancer.” *Journal of Personality and Social Psychology* 100 (2011): 129–148.
Exline, Julie J. and Ephraim D. Rose. “Religious and spiritual struggles.” In *Handbook of the Psychology of Religion and Spirituality*, edited by Raymond F. Paloutzian and Crystal L. Park, 315–330. New York: Guilford, 2013.
Exline, Julie J. and Ephraim D. Rose. “Religious and spiritual struggles.” In *Handbook of the Psychology of Religion and Spirituality*, edited by Raymond F. Paloutzian and Crystal L. Park, 380–398.
Exline, Julie J. and Erich D. Rose. “Religiöse und spirituelle Konflikte.” In *Religiosität: Die dunkle Seite: Beiträge zur empirischen Religionsforschung*, edited by Christian Zwingmann, Constantin Klein and Florian Jeserich, 65–90. Münster/New York: Waxmann, 2017.
Exline, Julie J., Ann Marie Yali and William C. Sanderson. “Guilt, Discord and Alienation: The Role of Religious Strain in Depression and Suicidality.” *Journal of Clinical Psychology* 56(2) (2000): 1481–1496.
Farooq, Saeed. “Collaborative care for depression: a literature review and a model for implementation in developing countries.” *International Health* 5(1) (2013): 24–28.
Fisher, Mickie L. and Julie J. Exline. “Moving toward self-forgiveness: Removing barriers related to shame, guilt, and regret.” *Social and Personality Psychology Compass* 4 (2010): 548–558.
Fitchett, George, Bruce D. Rybarczyk, Gail A. DeMarco and John J. Nicholas. “The role of religion in medical rehabilitation outcomes: A longitudinal study.” *Rehabilitation Psychology* 44 (1999): 1–22.
Fitchett, George, Urs Winter-Pfändler and Kenneth I. Pargament. “Struggle with the divine in Swiss patients visited by chaplains: prevalence and correlates.” *Journal of Health Psychology* 19(8) (2014): 966–976.

Folkman, Susan. "Positive psychological states and coping with severe stress." *Social Science & Medicine* 45 (1997): 1207–1221.
Francis, Leslie J., Harry M. Gibson and Mandy Robbins. "God images and self-worth among adolescents in Scotland." *Mental Health, Religion & Culture* 4(2) (2001): 103–108.
Frick, Eckhard. "Spiritual Care in der Humanmedizin: Profilierung und Vernetzung." In *Gesundheit – Religion – Spiritualität*, edited by Constantin Klein, Hendrik Berth and Friedrich Balck, 407–420. Weinheim: Beltz Juventa, 2011.
Frick, Eckhard, Klaus Baumann, Arndt Büssing, Christoph Jacobs and Jochen Sautermeister. "Spirituelle Trockenheit – Krise oder Chance? Am Beispiel der römisch-katholischen Priesterausbildung." *Wege zum Menschen* 70(1) (2018): 61–77.
Frick, Eckhard, Isgard Ohls, Gabriele Stotz-Ingenlath and Michael Utsch, eds. *Fallbuch Spiritualität in Psychotherapie und Psychiatrie*. Göttingen: Vandenhoeck & Ruprecht, 2018.
Frick, Eckard, Carola Riedner, Martin J. Fegg, S. Haufand and Gian D. Borasio. "A clinical interview assessing cancer patients' spiritual needs and preferences." *European Journal of Cancer Care* 15(3) (2006): 238–243.
Frick, Eckhard and Traugott Roser, eds. *Spiritualität und Medizin. Gemeinsame Sorge für den kranken Menschen*. Stuttgart: Kohlhammer, 2011.
Gall, Terry Lynn and Manal Guirguis-Younger. "Religious and spiritual coping: Current theory and research." In *APA Handbook of psychology, religion, and spirituality*, edited by Kenneth I. Pargament et al., 349–364. Washington, DC: American Psychological Association, 2013.
Geppert, Cynthia, Michael Bogenschutz and William Miller. "Development of a bibliography on religion, spirituality and addictions." *Drug and Alcohol Review* 26 (2007): 389–395.
Gilbert, Binford W. *The Pastoral Care of Depression: A Guidebook*. New York: Routledge, 2014.
Gräb, Wilhelm. *Lebensgeschichten – Lebensentwürfe – Sinndeutungen. Eine Praktische Theologie gelebter Religion*. Gütersloh: Gütersloher Verlagshaus, ²2000.
Gräb, Wilhelm. *Religion als Deutung des Lebens. Perspektiven einer Praktischen Theologie gelebter Religion*. Gütersloh: Gütersloher Verlagshaus, 2006.
Greenberg, Leslie S. and Jeanne C. Watson. *Emotion-focused therapy for depression*. Washington DC: American Psychological Association, 2006.
Greenway, Philip A., Lisa C. Milne and Veronica Clarke. "Personality variables, self-esteem and depression and an individual's perception of God." *Mental Health, Religion & Culture* 6(1) (2003): 45–58.
Grom, Bernhard. *Religionspsychologie*. München/Göttingen: Kösel-Verlag, 1992.
Grom, Bernhard. "Gesundheit und ‚Glaubensfaktor'. Religiosität als Komplementärmedizin?" *Stimmen der Zeit* 216 (1998): 413–424.
Grom, Bernhard. "Suizidalität und Religiosität." In *Suizidforschung und Suizidprävention am Ende des 20. Jahrhunderts. Theologische, epidemiologische, ökonomische, therapeutische Aspekte*, edited by Manfred Wolfersdorf and Christoph Franke, 19–35. Regensburg: Roderer, 2000.
Grom, Bernhard. "Wie froh macht die Frohbotschaft? Religiosität, subjektives Wohlbefinden und psychische Gesundheit." *Wege zum Menschen* 54 (2002): 196–204.
Grom, Bernhard. "Religiosität – psychische Gesundheit – subjektives Wohlbefinden: Ein Forschungsüberblick." In *Religiosität: Messverfahren und Studien zu Gesundheit und Lebensqualität. Neue Beiträge zur Religionspsychologie*, edited by Christian Zwingmann and Helfried Moosbrugger, 187–214. Münster: Waxmann, 2004.

Grossarth-Maticek, Ronald. *Selbstregulation, Autonomie und Gesundheit*. Berlin/New York: De Gruyter, 2003.

Gureje, Oye, Victor O. Lasebikan VO, Olusola Ephraim-Oluwanuga, Benjamin O. Olley and Lola Kola. "Community study of knowledge of and attitude to mental illness in Nigeria." *The British Journal of Psychiatry* 186 (2005): 436–441.

Gysels, Marjolein and Irene J. Higginson. *Improving supportive and palliative care for adults with cancer. Research evidence*. London: National Institute for Clinical Excellence, 2004.

Hackney, Charles H. and Glenn S. Sanders. "Religiosity and mental health: A meta-analysis of recent studies." *Journal for the Scientific Study of Religion* 42 (2003): 43–55.

Hamman, Jaco J. "Down and can't get up again: Serious depression." In *The Church Leader's Counseling Resource Book: A Guide to Mental Health and Social Problems*, edited by Cynthia Franklin and Rowena Fong, 154–163. Oxford: Oxford University Press, 2011.

Hanlon, Charlotte, Dawit Wondimagegn and Atalay Alem. "Lessons learnt in developing community mental health care in Africa." *World Psychiatry* 9 (2010): 185–189.

Hartmann, Fritz. "Krank oder bedingt gesund?" *Medizin Mensch Gesellschaft* 11 (1986): 170–179.

Hasenfratz, Hans-Peter. *Religion – was ist das?* Freiburg: Herder, 2002.

Hauschildt, Eberhard. *Alltagsseelsorge. Eine sozio-linguistische Analyse des pastoralen Geburtstagsbesuches*. Göttingen: Vandenhoeck & Ruprecht 1996.

Hauschildt, Eberhard. "Auf dem Weg zu einer Praktischen Theologie der Ehrenamtlichen-Seelsorge. Eine Skizze." *Pastoraltheologie* 99 (2010): 116–127.

Hauschildt, Eberhard. "'Spiritual Care' – eine Herausforderung für die Seelsorge?" *Materialdienst der EZW* 3 (2013): 83–90.

Haußmann, Annette. Ambivalenz und Dynamik. Religion in der häuslichen Pflege. Berlin: De Gruyter, 2019.

Haußmann, Annette. "Empirische Ergebnisse aus der Online-Umfrage unter Pfarrerinnen und Pfarrern." In *Menschen mit Depression*, edited by Birgit Weyel et al., 45–52. Gütersloh: Gütersloher Verlagshaus, 2014.

Haußmann, Annette. "Suche nach Spiritualität und Sinn bei Depression. Was können Seelsorge und Kognitive Verhaltenstherapie voneinander lernen?" In Spiritualität und Sinn. Seelsorge und Kognitive Verhaltenstherapie im Dialog, edited by Annette Haußmann and Rainer Höfelschweiger. Leipzig: Evangelische Verlagsanstalt, 2020 (in press).

Haußmann, Annette. "Suizidalität und Depression." In *Menschen mit Depression*, edited by Birgit Weyel et al., 36–44. Gütersloh: Gütersloher Verlagshaus, 2014.

Haußmann, Annette. "Wege zur Veränderung: Motivierende Gesprächsführung." In *Das Depressions-Buch für Pflege- und Gesundheitsberufe: Menschen mit Depressionen gekonnt pflegen und behandeln*, edited by Thomas Hax-Schoppenhorst and Stefan Jünger, 269–281. Bern: Hogrefe, 2016.

Haußmann, Annette. "Einsamkeit und Spiritualität." In *Das Einsamkeitsbuch. Wie Gesundheitsberufe einsame Menschen verstehen, unterstützen und integrieren können*, edited by Thomas Hax-Schoppenhorst, 153–163. Bern: Hogrefe, 2018.

Haußmann, Annette and Friedemann Bresch. "Seelsorgerliche Gesprächsführung mit depressiven Menschen." In *Menschen mit Depression*, edited by Birgit Weyel et al., 179–194. Gütersloh: Gütersloher Verlagshaus, 2014.

Hayward, David R., Amy D. Owen, Harold G. Koenig, David C. Steffens and Martha E. Payne. "Longitudinal relationships of religion with posttreatment depression severity in older psychiatric patients: Evidence of direct and indirect effects." *Depression research and treatment* (2012): 1–8.

Hayward, Richard D. and Neal Krause. "Trajectories of late-life change in God-mediated control." *The journals of gerontology. Series B, Psychological sciences and social sciences* 68(1) (2013): 49–58.

Hefti, René. "Spiritualität und Medizin. Ein empirischer Beitrag zur Spiritualitätsforschung." In *Spiritualität im Diskurs. Spiritualitätsforschung in theologischer Perspektive*, edited by Ralph Kunz and Claudia Kohli Reichenbach, 241–261. Zürich: Theologischer Verlag Zürich, 2012.

Hell, Daniel. "Psychodynamik der Depression und Achtsamkeit." In *Dunkle Nacht und Depression: Geistliche und psychische Krisen verstehen und unterscheiden*, edited by Regina Bäumer and Michael Plattig, 10–21. Ostfildern: Grünewald, 2008.

Henning, Christian. "Die Geschichte der Religionspsychologie im deutschsprachigen Raum." In *Einführung in die Religionspsychologie*, edited by Christian Henning, Sebastian Murken and Erich Nestler, 9–90. Paderborn: Schöningh, 2003.

Hermelink, Jan, Ingrid Lukatis and Monika Wohlrab-Sahr. *Kirche in der Vielfalt der Lebensbezüge. Die vierte EKD-Erhebung über Kirchenmitgliedschaft*, Vol. 2, *Analysen zu Gruppendiskussionen und Erzählinterviews*. Gütersloh: Gütersloher Verlagshaus, 2006.

Higgins, Nancy, C. Alec Pollard and William T. Merkel. "Relationship between religion-related factors and obsessive compulsive disorder." *Current Psychology* 11 (1992): 79–85.

Hirsch, Jameson K., Jon R. Webb and Elizabeth L. Jeglic. "Forgiveness, depression, and suicidal behavior among a diverse sample of college students." *Journal of Clinical Psychology* 67(9) (2011): 896–906.

Hodapp, Bastian. *Religiosität/Spiritualität und psychische Gesundheit – eine Metaanalyse über Studien aus dem deutschsprachigen Raum*. Hamburg: Kovač, 2017.

Hodapp, Bastian and Christian Zwingmann. "Religiosity/Spirituality and mental health: a meta-analysis of studies from the German-speaking area." *Journal of Religion and Health* 58 (2019): 1970–1998.

Hoff, Andreas et al. "Religion and reduced cancer risk – What is the explanation? A review." *European Journal of Cancer Care* 17 (2008): 2573–2579.

Hoffmann, Mirjam. *Religiosität und psychische Gesundheit*. Stuttgart: Kohlhammer, 2019.

Holloway, Margret, Sue Adamson, Wilf McSherry and John Swinton. *Spiritual care at the end of life: A systematic review of the literature*. Hull: University of Hull, Department of Health, 2011.

Holt, Cheryl L., David L. Roth, Jin Huang and Eddie M. Clark. "Role of religious social support in longitudinal relationships between religiosity and health-related outcomes in African Americans." *Journal of Behavioral Medicine* 41(1) (2018): 62–73.

Huber, Stefan. *Dimensionen der Religiosität: Skalen, Messmodelle und Ergebnisse einer empirisch orientierten Religionspsychologie*. Bern/Göttingen: Huber, 1996.

Huber, Stefan. *Zentralität und Inhalt: Ein neues multidimensionales Messmodell der Religiosität*. Opladen: Leske & Budrich, 2003.

Huber, Stefan. "Religiosität in Deutschland, Österreich und der Schweiz." In *Gesundheit – Religion – Spiritualität*, edited by Constantin Klein, Hendrik Berth and Friedrich Balck, 163–187. Weinheim: Beltz Juventa, 2011.

Huber, Stefan, Mathias Allemand and Odilo W. Huber. "Forgiveness by God and Human Forgivingness: The Centrality of the Religiosity Makes the Difference." *Archive for the Psychology of Religion* 33(1) (2011): 115–134.

Huber, Stefan, and Odilo W. Huber. "The Centrality of Religiosity Scale (CRS)." *Religions* 3 (2012): 710–724.

Huber, Stefan, and Constantin Klein. "Spirituelle und religiöse Konstrukträume." In *Spiritualität transdisziplinär. Wissenschaftliche Grundlagen im Zusammenhang mit Gesundheit und Krankheit*, edited by Arndt Büssing and Niko Kohls, 53–66. Berlin/ Heidelberg: Springer-Verlag, 2011.

Illich, Ivan. *Nemesis der Medizin*. Reinbek: Rowohlt, 1977.

Ingram, Rick E. and Joseph M. Price, *Vulnerability to psychopathology. Risk across the lifespan*. New York: Guilford, 2001.

Jakob, Beate and Peter Bartmann. "Gesundheit und Gesundheitsförderung. Ansätze zu einer Integration der spirituellen Dimension in Konzepte und die Arbeit der WHO." In *Spiritualität und seelische Gesundheit*, edited by J. Armbruster et al., 48–62. Köln: Psychiatrie Verlag, 2013.

Jakob, Beate. "Bibelarbeit zum Thema Depression." In *Menschen mit Depression*, edited by Birgit Weyel and Beate Jakob, 128–139. Gütersloh: Gütersloher Verlagshaus, 2014.

Jim, Heather S. et al. "Religion, spirituality, and physical health in cancer patients: A meta-analysis," *Cancer* 121 (2015): 3760–3768.

Kabat-Zinn, Jon. "Mindfulness-based interventions in context: Past, present, and future." *Clinical Psychology: Science and Practice* 10 (2003): 144–156.

Kaiser, Peter. "Pathologische Religiosität im psychiatrischen Kontext." In *Religiosität: Die dunkle Seite: Beiträge zur empirischen Religionsforschung*, edited by Christian Zwingmann, Constantin Klein and Florian Jeserich, 227–252. Münster/New York: Waxmann, 2017.

Kalish, Naomi. "Evidence-based spiritual care: A literature review." *Current Opinion in Supportive and Palliative Care* 6 (2012): 242–246.

Kanth, Vandana. *Duncan Hospital, Community Health and Development Programme, Needs assessment on domestic violence in Raxaul Block* (unpublished study, 2011).

Karle, Isolde. "Die Sehnsucht nach Heil und nach Heilung in der kirchlichen Praxis." In *Krankheitsdeutung in der postsäkularen Gesellschaft*, edited by Günter Thomas and Isolde Karle, 543–556. Stuttgart: Kohlhammer, 2009.

Kauye, Felix et al. "Increasing the capacity of health surveillance assistants in community mental health care in a developing country, Malawi." *Malawi Medical Journal* 23(3) (2011): 85.

Kauye, Felix, Rachel Jenkins and Atif Rahman. "Training primary health care workers in mental health and its impact on diagnosis of common mental disorders in primary care of a developing country, Malawi: a cluster-randomized controlled trial." *Psychological Medicine* 44(3) (2014): 657–666.

Kendler, Kenneth S., Charles O. Gardner and Carol A. Prescott. "Clarifying the relationship between religiosity and psychiatric illness: The impact of covariates and the specificity of buffering effects." *Twin Research and Human Genetics* 2 (1999): 137–144.

Kennedy, Gary J. "Religion and Depression." In *Handbook of Religion and mental health*, edited by Harold G. Koenig, 130–145. San Diego: Academic Press, 1998.

Kießling, Klaus. *Seelsorge bei Seelenfinsternis*. Freiburg: Herder, 2002.

Kirkpatrick, Lee A. *Attachment, evolution, and the psychology of religion*. New York: Guilford, 2004.

Klein, Constantin and Cornelia Albani, "Religiosität und psychische Gesundheit – empirische Befunde und Erklärungsansätze." In *Gesundheit – Religion – Spiritualität*, edited by Constantin Klein, Hendrik Berth and Friedrich Balck, 215–245. Weinheim: Beltz Juventa, 2011.

Klein, Constantin and Cornelia Albani. "Die Bedeutung von Religion für die psychische Befindlichkeit: Mögliche Erklärungsansätze und allgemeines Wirkmodell." *Zeitschrift für Nachwuchswissenschaftler* 3 (2011): 7–58.

Klein, Constantin, Hendrik Berth and Friedrich Balck, eds. *Gesundheit – Religion – Spiritualität: Konzepte, Befunde und Erklärungsansätze*. Weinheim: Beltz Juventa, 2011.

Klein, Constantin, Sonja Gottschling and Christian Zwingmann. "Deutschsprachige Fragebögen zur Messung von Religiosität/Spiritualität. Ein empirisch gestützter Vergleich ausgewählter Skalen." *Spiritual Care* 1(3) (2012): 22–35

Klessmann, Michael. "Macht und Ohnmacht in Seelsorge und Beratung." *Wege zum Menschen* 67 (2015): 344–357.

Klessmann, Michael. *Pastoralpsychologische Perspektiven in der Seelsorge: Grenzgänge zwischen Theologie und Psychologie*. Göttingen: Vandenhoeck & Ruprecht, 2017.

Klosinksi, Gunther, ed. *Religion als Chance oder Risiko*. Bern: Verlag Hans Huber, 1994.

Knieps, Franz, and Holger Pfaff, eds. *Gesundheit und Arbeit. Zahlen, Daten, Fakten*. BKK Gesundheitsreport 2016. Berlin: Medizinisch Wissenschaftliche Verlagsgesellschaft, 2016.

Koch, Stefanie. "Wie können Kirchengemeinden depressiv kranke Menschen und ihre Angehörigen unterstützen? Interviews mit ausgewählten Personengruppen." In *Menschen mit Depression*, edited by Birgit Weyel et al., 53–97. Gütersloh: Gütersloher Verlagshaus, 2014.

Koenig, Harold G. *Is Religion Good for your Health?* New York/London: Haworth Pastoral Press, 1997.

Koenig, Harold G. *Spirituality in patient care: Why, how, when and what*. Philadelphia: Templeton Foundation Press, 2002.

Koenig, Harold G. "Concerns about measuring 'spirituality' in research." *Journal of Nervous and Mental Disease* 196 (2008): 349–355.

Koenig, Harold and Raphael Bonelli. "Mental disorders, religion and spirituality 1990 to 2010: a systematic evidence based review." *Journal of Religion and Health* 52 (2013): 657–673.

Koenig, Harold G., Dana King and Verna B. Carson. *Handbook of religion and health*. 2nd edition. New York: Oxford University Press, 2012.

Koenig, Harold G. and David B. Larson. "Religion and mental health. Evidence for an association." *International Review of Psychiatry* 13 (2001): 67–78.

Koenig, Harold G., Michael E. McCullough and David B. Larson, *Handbook of religion and health*. New York: Oxford University Press, 2001.

Kozasa, Elisa H., Ruth F. Santos, Adriana D. Rueda and Ana A. Benedito-Silva et al. "Evaluation of Siddha Samadhi Yoga for anxiety and depression symptoms: A preliminary study." *Psychological Reports* 103 (2008): 271–274.

Krahl, Wolfgang. "Mental Health in Developing Countries – Global Mental Health. 4th International Symposium 10th November 2012. Munich." *Curare* 36 (2013): 144–147.

Kramer, Teresa L., Dean Blevins et al. "Ministers' perceptions of depression: A model to understand and improve care." *Journal of Religion and Health* 46(1) (2007): 123–139.

Kramer, Teresa L., Dean Blevins, Terri L. Miller, Martha M. Phillips, Vanessa Davis and Billy Burris. "Ministers' perceptions of depression: A model to understand and improve care." *Journal of Religion and Health* 46(1) (2007): 123–139.

Krause, Neal and David R. Hayward. "Social Factors in the Church and Positive Religious Coping Responses: Assessing Differences Among Older Whites, Older Blacks, and Older Mexican Americans." *Review of Religious Research* 54(4) (2012): 519–541.

Krause, Neil M. and Keith M. Wulff. "Friendship Ties in the Church and Depressive Symptoms: Exploring Variations by Age." *Review of Religious Research* 46 (2005): 325–340.

Kuckartz, Udo. *Einführung in die computergestützte Analyse qualitativer Daten*. Wiesbaden: VS Verlag für Sozialwissenschaften, ^{3}2010.

Kuckartz, Udo. *Qualitative Inhaltsanalyse. Methoden, Praxis, Computerunterstützung*. Weinheim and Basel: Beltz Juventa, ^{2}2014.

Kunz, Ralph. "Beten in der Anfechtung." In *Gebet als Resonanzereignis. Annäherungen im Horizont von Spiritual Care*, edited by Simon Peng-Keller, 159–192. Göttingen: Vandenhoeck & Ruprecht, 2017.

Küpper, Beate and Andreas Zick. "Riskanter Glaube. Religiosität und Abwertung." In *Deutsche Zustände. Folge 4*, edited by Wilhelm Heitmeyer, 179–188. Frankfurt: Suhrkamp, 2006.

Lammer, Kerstin. *Wie Seelsorge wirkt*. Stuttgart: Kohlhammer-Verlag, 2020.

Lawler-Row, Kathleen A. "Forgiveness as a mediator of the religiosity-health relationship." *Psychology of Religion and Spirituality* 2 (2010): 1–16.

Lazarus, Richard S. and Susan Folkman. *Stress, appraisal, and coping*. New York: Springer, 1984.

Liedke, Ulf. "Menschen. Leben. Vielfalt." *Pastoraltheologie* 101 (2012): 71–86.

Lindner, Judith. "Einflüsse von Religiosität und Vergebung auf die psychische Gesundheit." *Wege zum Menschen* 68 (2016): 360–371.

Louw, Daniël. "'Verbing God' within the dynamics of 'Lived Religion'. 'Sympathetic Rites of Passage' in a Practical Theological approach to the complexity of everyday life." In *Pluralisation and social change. Dynamics of lived religion in South Africa and in Germany*. Praktische Theologie im Wissenschaftsdiskurs 21, edited by Lars Charbonnier, Johan Cilliers, Matthias Mader, Cas Wepener and Birgit Weyel, 51–65. Berlin: De Gruyter, 2018.

Luhtanen, Riia K. and Jennifer Crocker. "Alcohol use in college students: Effects of level of self-esteem, narcissism and contingencies of self-worth." *Psychology and Addictive Behaviors* 19 (2005): 99–103.

Luther, Henning. "Wahrnehmen und Ausgrenzen oder die doppelte Verdrängung. Zur Tradition des seelsorgerlich-diakonischen Blicks," *Theologia Practica* 23 (1988): 250–266

Luz, Ulrich. *Evangelisch-Katholischer Kommentar zum Neuen Testament*. Tb. 2, *Das Evangelium nach Matthäus (Mt 8–17)*. Zürich/Neukirchen: Benzinger/Neukirchener, 1990.

Martin, Alice M. *Exploring Forgiveness: The Relationship Between Feeling Forgiven by God and Self-Forgiveness for an Interpersonal Offense*. Electronic Thesis, 2008.

Maselko, Joana et al. "Religious service attendance and allostatic load among high-functioning elderly." *Psychosomatic Medicine* 69 (2007): 464–472.

Maselko, Joanna, R. David Hayward, Alexandra Hanlon, Stephen Buka and Keith Meador. "Religious service attendance and major depression: A case of reverse causality?" *American Journal of Epidemiology* 175(6) (2012): 576–583.

Matthews, Dale A. et al. "Religious commitment and health status: A review of the research and implications for family medicine." *Archives of Family Medicine* 7 (1998): 118–124.

Mayer-Scheu, Josef, and Rudolf Kautsky, eds. *Vom Behandeln zum Heilen. Die vergessene Dimension im Krankenhaus*. Wien/Göttingen: Herder, 1980.

McClintock, Clayton H., Micheline Anderson, Connie Svob et al. "Multidimensional understanding of religiosity/spirituality: relationship to major depression and familial risk." *Psychological Medicine* (2018): 1–10.

McCullough, Michael E. "Research on religion-accomodative counseling: Review and meta-analysis." *Journal of Counseling Psychology* 46 (1999): 92–98.

McCullough, Michael E., Kenneth I. Pargament and Carl E. Thoresen, eds., *Forgiveness. Theory, research, and practice.* New York: Guilford, 2000.

McCullough, Michael E., Robert A. Emmons and Jo-Ann Tsang. "The grateful disposition: A conceptual and empirical topography." *Journal of Personality and Social Psychology* 82 (2002): 112–127.

McCullough, Michael E., William T. Hoyt, David B. Larson, Harold G. Koenig and Carl Thoresen. "Religious involvement and mortality: A meta-analytic review." *Health Psychology* 19 (2000): 211–222.

McIntosh, Daniel. "Religion as a schema, with implications for the relation between religion and coping." *International Journal for the Psychology of Religion* 5 (1995): 1–16.

Miller, Lisa, Priva Wickramaratne, Marc J. Gameroff, Mia Sage, Craig E. Tenke and Myrna M. Weissman. "Religiosity and major depression in adults at high risk: A ten-year prospective study." *The American Journal of Psychiatry* 169(1) (2012): 89–94.

Mohr, Sylvia, Christiane Gilliéron, Laurence Borras, Pierre-Yves Brandt and Philippe Huguelet. "The assessment of spirituality and religiousness in schizophrenia." *Journal of Nervous and Mental Disease* 195 (2007): 247–253.

Moosbrugger, Helfried, Christian Zwingmann and Dirk Frank. "Psychologische Aspekte von Religiosität." In *Religiosität, Persönlichkeit und Verhalten. Beiträge zur Religionspsychologie*, edited by Helfried Moosbrugger, Christian Zwingmann an Dirk Frank, 3–8. Münster: Waxmann, 1996.

Moran, Michael, Kevin J. Flannelly, Andrew J. Weaver, Jon A. Overvold, Winfried Hess and Jo Clare Wilson. "A study of pastoral care, referral, and consultation practices among clergy in four settings in the New York City area." *Pastoral Psychology* 53(3) (2005): 255–265.

Moran, Michael, Kevin J. Flannelly et al. "A study of pastoral care, referral, and consultation practices among clergy in four settings in the New York City area." *Pastoral Psychology* 53(3) (2005): 255–266.

Morgenthaler, Christoph. *Systemische Seelsorge.* Stuttgart: Kohlhammer, 1999.

Morgenthaler, Christoph. *Seelsorge.* Lehrbuch Praktische Theologie 3. Gütersloh: Gütersloher Verlagshaus, 2009.

Moriarty, Glendon. *Pastoral Care of Depression: Helping clients heal their relationship with God.* Binghamton: Routledge, 2006.

Moser, Tilman. *Gottesvergiftung.* Frankfurt am Main: Suhrkamp, 1976.

Mueller, Paul S., David J. Plevak and Teresa A. Rummans. "Religious involvement, spirituality, and medicine: Implications for clinical practice." *Mayo Clinic Proceedings* 76 (2001): 1225–1235.

Murken, Sebastian. "Ungesunde Religiosität – Entscheidungen der Psychologie?" In *Kritik an Religionen*, edited by Gritt Maria Klinkhammer, Steffen Rink and Tobias Frick, 157–172. Marburg: Diagonal-Verlag, 1997.

Murken, Sebastian. *Gottesbeziehung und psychische Gesundheit. Die Entwicklung eines Modells und seine empirische Überprüfung.* Münster: Waxmann, 1998.

Murken, Sebastian. "Das Konzept der Zwölf Schritte und der ‚Höheren Macht'. Zum Genesungsprogramm der Anonymen Alkoholiker." *Prävention* 31 (2008): 57–60.

Murken, Sebastian, Katja Möschl, Claudia Müller and Claudia Appel. "Entwicklung und Validierung der Skalen zur Gottesbeziehung und zum religiösen Coping." In *Spiritualität transdisziplinär: Wissenschaftliche Grundlagen im Zusammenhang mit Gesundheit und Krankheit*, edited by Arndt Büssing and Niko Kohls, 75–90. Berlin: Springer, 2011.

Murray, Kelly and Joseph W. Ciarrocchi. "The dark side of Religion, Spirituality and the moral emotions: shame, guilt, and negative religiosity as markers for life dissatisfaction." *Journal of Pastoral Counseling* 42 (2007): 22–41.

Nauer, Doris. *Spiritual Care statt Seelsorge?* Stuttgart: Kohlhammer, 2015.

Neeleman, Jan and Glenn Lewis. "Suicide, religion, and socioeconomic conditions. An ecological study in 26 countries." *Journal of Epidemiology and Community Health* 53 (1999): 204–210.

Ness, Peter H. and David B. Larson. "Religion, Senescence, and Mental Health." *American Journal of Geriatric Psychiatry* 10(4) (2002): 386–397.

Norton, Maria C., Archana Singh and Ingmar Skoog. "Church attendance and new episodes of major depression in a community study of older adults: The Cache County Study." *The journals of gerontology / B* 63(3) (2008): 129–137.

Noth, Isabelle and Jessica Lampe. "Spiritual Struggles." In: Encyclopedia of Psychology and Religion, edited by David A. Leeming (Berlin / Heidelberg: Springer, 2019), 1–4.

Noth, Isabelle, Emanuel Schweizer and Georg Wenz, eds. *Pastoral and spiritual care across religions and cultures: Seelsorge und Spiritual Care in interkultureller Perspektive.* Göttingen/Bristol: Vandenhoeck & Ruprecht, 2017.

Oman, Douglas and Dwayne Reed. "Religion and mortality among the community-dwelling elderly." *American Journal of Public Health* 88 (1998): 1469–1475.

Paloutzian, Raymond F. and Crystal L. Park, eds. *Handbook of the Psychology of Religion and Spirituality.* New York: Guilford, 2005.

Pardini, Dustin, Thomas G. Plante and Allen C. Sherman. "Strength of religious faith and its association with mental health outcomes among recovering alcoholics and addicts." *Journal of Substance Abuse Treatment* 19 (2001): 347–354.

Parenteau, Stacy C., Nancy A. Hamilton, Wei Wu, Kevin Latinis, Lori B. Waxenberg and Mary Y. Brinkmeyer. "The mediating role of secular coping strategies in the relationship between religious appraisals and adjustment to chronic pain: The middle road to Damascus." *Social Indicators Research* 104 (2011): 407–425.

Pargament, Kenneth I. "Religion and the Problem-Solving Process: Three Styles of Coping." *Journal for the Scientific Study of Religion* 27(1) (1988): 90–104.

Pargament, Kenneth I. *The psychology of religion and coping. Theory, research, practice.* New York: Guilford, 1997.

Pargament, Kenneth I. *Spiritually integrated psychotherapy: Understanding and addressing the sacred.* New York: Guilford Press, 2007.

Pargament, Kenneth I., Gene G. Ano and Amy B. Wachholtz. "The religious dimensions of coping: Advances in theory, research, and practice." In *Handbook of the Psychology of Religion and Spirituality*, edited by Raymond F. Paloutzian and Crystal L. Park, 479–495. New York: Guilford, 2005.

Pargament, Kenneth I., Julia J. Exline and James W. Jones, eds. *APA Handbook of psychology, religion, and spirituality*, Vol 1, *Context, theory, and research*. Washington, DC: American Psychological Association, 2013.

Pargament, Kenneth I., Melissa D. Falb, Gene G. Ano and Amy B. Wachholtz. "The Religious Dimensions of Coping: Advances in Theory, Research, and Practice." In *Handbook of the Psychology of Religion and Spirituality*, edited by Raymond F. Paloutzian and Crystal L. Park, 560–579. New York, Guilford, 2013.

Pargament, Kenneth I., Harold G. Koenig, Nalini Tarakeshwar and June Hahn. "Religious struggle as a predictor of mortality among medically ill elderly patients: A two-year longitudinal study." *Archives of Internal Medicine* 161 (2001): 1881–1885.

Pargament, Kenneth I., Harold G. Koenig, Nalini Tarakeshwar and June Hahn. "Religious Coping Methods as Predictors of Psychological, Physical and Spiritual Outcomes among Medically Ill Elderly Patients: A Two-year Longitudinal Study." *Journal of Health Psychology* 9(6) (2004): 713–730.

Pargament, Kenneth I., Annette Mahoney, Julie J. Exline, James W. Jones and Edward P. Shafranske. "Envisioning an integrative paradigm for the psychology of religion and spirituality." In *APA Handbook of Psychology, Religion, and Spirituality*, edited by Kenneth I. Pargament et al., 3–19. Washington, DC: American Psychological Association, 2013.

Park, Crystal L. and Jeanne M. Slattery. "Religion, Spirituality, and Mental Health." In *Handbook of the Psychology of Religion and Spirituality*, edited by Raymond F. Paloutzian and Crystal L. Park, 540–559. New York: Guilford, 2005.

Patel, Vikram and Martin Prince. "Global Mental Health: a new global health field comes of age." *JAMA* 303/19 (2010): 1976–1977.

Payne, Jennifer. "The influence of secular and theological education on pastors' depression intervention decisions." *Journal of Religion and Health* 53(5) (2014): 1398–1413.

Pearce, Michelle J. et al. "Unmet spiritual care needs impact emotional and spiritual well-being." *Supportive Care in Cancer* 20 (2012): 2269–2276.

Peng-Keller, Simon. "Spiritual Care im Gesundheitswesen des 20. Jahrhunderts. Von der sozialen Medizin zur WHO-Diskussion im die 'spirituelle Dimension'." In *Spiritual Care im globalisierten Gesundheitswesen. Historische Hintergründe und aktuelle Entwicklungen*, edited by S. Peng-Keller and D. Neuhold, 13–72. Darmstadt: Wissenschaftliche Buchgesellschaft, 2019.

Pérez, John E., Amy R. Smith, Rebecca L. Norris, Katia M. Canenguez, Elizabeth F. Tracey and Susan B. DeCristofaro. "Types of prayer and depressive symptoms among cancer patients: The mediating role of rumination and social support." *Journal of Behavioral Medicine* 34(6) (2011): 519–530.

Peteet, John R. "Spiritually integrated treatment of depression: A conceptual framework." *Depression Research and Treatment* (2012): 1–6.

Peteet, John R. *Depression and the soul: A guide to Spiritually integrated Treatment*. New York: Routledge, 2010.

Petts, R. T. and Anne Joliff. "Religion and Adolescent Depression: The Impact of Race and Gender." *Review of Religious Research* 49(4) (2008): 395–414.

Pfeifer, Samuel. "Seelenfinsternis und dunkle Nacht der Seele – Depression und Spiritualität." In *Psychotherapie und Spiritualität: Mit existenziellen Konflikten und Transzendenzfragen professionell umgehen*, edited by Michael Utsch, Raphael M. Bonelli and Samuel Pfeifer, 121–132. Berlin/Heidelberg: Springer, 2014.

Phillips, R.L. and D.A. Snowdon. "Association of meat and coffee use with cancers of the large bowel, breast, and prostate among Seventh-Day Adventists: Preliminary results." *Cancer Research* 43 (5 Suppl.) (1983): 2403–2408.

Pieper, Joseph Z.T. “Religious coping in highly religious inpatients.” *Mental Health, Religion & Culture* 7 (2004): 349–363.

Plante, Thomas G. and Naveen K. Sharma. “Religious faith and mental health outcomes.” In *Faith and health. Psychological perspectives*, edited by Thomas G. Plante and Allen C. Sherman, 240–261. New York: Guilford, 2001.

Puchalski, Christina, and Anna Romer. “Taking a spiritual history allows clinicians to understand patients more fully.” *Journal of Palliative Medicine* 3 (2000): 129–137

Puchalski, Christina. “Spiritual Care: Practical tools.” In *A time for listening and caring: Spirituality and the care of the chronically ill and dying*, edited by Christina Puchalski, 229–251. Oxford/New York: Oxford University Press, 2006.

Raphael, Frances J., Shashi Rani, R. Bale and Lynne M. Drummond. “Religion, ethnicity and obsessive-compulsive disorder.” *International Journal of Social Psychiatry* 42 (1996): 38–44.

Reicherzer, Markus. *Depressive Störungen: Differentielle manualisierte Behandlung mit Skillstraining und Psychoedukation*. Stuttgart: Schattauer GmbH Verlag für Medizin und Naturwissenschaften, 2017.

Reischies, Friedel M. “Religiös-spirituelle Dimension bei psychischen Krankheiten – Depression: Positive und negative Auswirkungen religiösen Erlebens.” *Spiritual Care* 6 (2017): 31–35.

Riedner, Carola and Thomas Hagen. “Spirituelle Anamnese.” In *Spiritualität und Medizin. Gemeinsame Sorge für den kranken Menschen*. Münchner Reihe Palliative Care 4, edited by Eckhard Frick and Traugott Roser, 234–241. Stuttgart ^{2}2011.

Riffer, Friedrich, Elmar Kaiser, Manuel Sprung and Lore Streibl, eds. *Das Fremde: Flucht – Trauma – Resilienz. Aktuelle traumaspezifische Konzepte in der Psychosomatik. Psychosomatik im Zentrum*. Berlin/Heidelberg: Springer, 2018.

Ritschl, Dietrich. “Gesundheit: Gnade oder Rechtsanspruch.” In *Konzepte. Ökumene, Medizin, Ethik*, edited by Dietrich Ritschl, 266–271. München: Kaiser, 1986.

Ritschl, Dietrich. “Was ist der Mensch – in Krankheit und Gesundheit? Anthropologische Ansätze verschiedener Krankheits- und Gesundheitsverständnisse.” *Wege zum Menschen* 51 (1999): 396–410.

Ritter, Werner Heinz. “Heilung, Energie, Geist als wissenschaftliche Herausforderung.” In *Heilung – Energie – Geist. Heilung zwischen Wissenschaft, Religion und Geschäft*, edited by Werner Heinz Ritter and Bernhard Wolf, 15–30. Göttingen: Vandenhoeck & Ruprecht, 2005.

Rogers, Carl R. Therapeut und Klient. Grundlagen der Gesprächspsychotherapie. München: Kindler, 1977.

Roleder, Felix and Birgit Weyel. *Vernetzte Kirchengemeinde. Persönliche Beziehungen, religiöse Kommunikation, kirchliche Geselligkeit und zivilgesellschaftliche Beteiligung. Analysen zur Gesamtnetzwerkerhebung der V. Kirchenmitgliedschaftsuntersuchung der EKD*. Leipzig: Evangelische Verlagsanstalt 2019.

Roser, Traugott. *Spiritual Care. Der Beitrag von Seelsorge zum Gesundheitswesen*, 391–398. Stuttgart: Kohlhammer, ^{2}2017.

Runnels, Ratonia C. and Mel Stauber. “Today’s best pastoral care: Church-based mental health and social programs.” In *The Church Leader’s Counseling Resource Book: A Guide to Mental Health and Social Problems*, edited by Cynthia Franklin and Rowena Fong, 431–448. Oxford: Oxford University Press, 2011.

Salsman, John M. et al. “A meta-analytic approach to examining the correlation between religion/spirituality and mental health in cancer.” *Cancer* 121 (2015): 3769–3778.

Sampath, Janani. “TNN.” *The Times of India* (Jan 20, 2014).

Sautermeister, Jochen and Tobias Skuban, eds. *Handbuch psychiatrisches Grundwissen für die Seelsorge*. Freiburg: Herder, 2018.

Saxena, Shekhar, Graham Thornicorft, Martin Knapp and Harvey Whiteford. "Global Mental Health, 2. Resources for mental health: scarcity, inequity, and inefficiency." *Lancet* 370 (2007): 878–889.

Schlenker, Jochen. "Zur Sprache bringen. Supervision mit Ehrenamtlichen in der Ausbildung zur Seelsorgerin, zum Seelsorger." *Wege zum Menschen* 66 (2014): 273–288.

Schlingensief, Christoph. "*So schön wie hier kanns im Himmel gar nicht sein!*" *Tagebuch einer Krebserkrankung*. Köln: Kiepenheuer & Witsch, 2009.

Schnabel, Ulrich. *Die Vermessung des Glaubens*, 2. Aufl. München: Blessing Verlag, 2010.

Schneidereit-Mauth, Heike. *Ressourcenorientierte Seelsorge. Salutogenese als Modell für seelsorgerliches Handeln*. Gütersloh: Gütersloher Verlagshaus, 2015.

Schnell, Tatjana. *Psychologie des Lebenssinns*. Berlin: Springer, 2016.

Schowalter, Marion and Sebastian Murken. "Religion und psychische Gesundheit – empirische Zusammenhänge komplexer Konstrukte." In *Einführung in die Religionspsychologie*, edited by Christian Henning, Sebastian Murken and Erich Nestler, 138–162. Paderborn: UTB, 2003.

Schult, Maike. "*Ein Hauch von Ordnung*". *Traumaarbeit als Aufgabe der Seelsorge*. Arbeiten zur Praktischen Theologie. Vol. 64. Leipzig: Evangelische Verlagsanstalt, 2020.

Schultz, Jessica M., Benjamin A. Tallman and Elizabeth M. Altmaier. "Pathways to posttraumatic growth: The contributions of forgiveness and importance of religion and spirituality." *Psychology of Religion and Spirituality* 2 (2010): 104–114.

Seidelmann, Stephan. *Evangelische engagiert – Tendenz steigend. Sonderauswertung des dritten Freiwilligensurveys für die Evangelische Kirche, Sozialwissenschaftliches Institut der EKD*. Hannover: EKD, 2012.

Shafranske, Edward P., ed. *Religion and the clinical practice of psychology*. Washington, DC: American Psychological Association, 1996.

Shafranske, Edward P. "The psychology of religion in clinical and counseling psychology." In *Handbook of the Psychology of Religion and Spirituality*, edited by Raymond F. Paloutzian and Crystal L. Park, 496–514. New York, Guilford, 2005.

Shapiro, Shauna L., Doug Oman, Carl E. Thoresen, Thomas G. Plante and Tim Flinders. "Cultivating mindfulness: Effects on well-being." *Journal of Clinical Psychology* 64 (2008): 840–862.

Sherman, Allen C. and Stephanie Simonton. "Spirituality and cancer." In *Spirit, science and health. How the spiritual mind fuels physical wellness*, edited by Thomas G. Plante and Carl E. Thoresen, 157–175. Westport, CT: Praeger, 2007.

Shor, Eran and David Roelfs. "The longevity effects of religious and nonreligious participation: A meta-analysis and meta-regression." *Journal for the Scientific Study of Religion* 52 (2013): 120–145.

Shreve-Neiger, Andrea K. and Barry A. Edelstein. "Religion and anxiety: A critical review of the literature." *Clinical Psychology Review* 24 (2004): 379–397.

Simonson, Julia, Claudia Vogel and Clemens Tesch-Römer, eds. *Freiwilliges Engagement in Deutschland. Der Deutsche Freiwilligensurvey 2014*. Berlin: Springer-Verlag, 2017.

Simonson, Julia, Claudia Vogel and Clemens Tesch-Römer, eds. *Tabellenanhang. Freiwilliges Engagement in Deutschland – Der Deutsche Freiwilligensurvey 2014*. Wiesbaden: Springer VS, 2016.

Smith, Timothy B., Michael E. McCullough and Justin Poll. "Religiousness and depression: Evidence for a main effect and the moderating influence of stressful life events." *Psychological Bulletin* 129(4) (2003): 614–636.

Stack, Steven. "Religiosity, depression, and suicide." In *Religion and mental health*, edited by John F. Schumaker, 87–98. Oxford/New York: Oxford University Press, 1992.

Stark, Rodney and Roger Finke. *Acts of faith: Explaining the human side of religion*. Berkeley, CA: University of California Press, 2000.

Steck, Wolfgang. "Der Ursprung der Seelsorge in der Alltagswelt." *Theologische Zeitschrift* 43 (1987): 175.

Stefanek, Michael, Paige G. McDonald and Stephanie A. Hess. "Religion, spirituality and cancer: Current status and methodological challenges." *Psycho-Oncology* 14 (2005): 450–463.

Stotz-Ingenlath, Gabriele and Eckard Frick. "Depressives Schulderleben: Symptomatologie und Diagnostik." *Schweizer Archiv für Neurologie und Psychiatrie* 157(3) (2006): 94–102.

Strawbridge, William J., Sarah J. Shema, Richard D. Cohen and George A. Kaplan. "Religious attendance increases survival by improving and maintaining good health practices, mental health, and stable marriages." *Annals of Behavioral Medicine* 23 (2001): 68–74.

Streib, Heinz et al. *Deconversion. Qualitative and quantitative results from cross-cultural research in Germany and the United States of America.* Göttingen: Vandenhoeck & Ruprecht, 2009.

Streib, Heinz and Constantin Klein. "Atheists, agnostics, and apostates." In *APA handbook of psychology, religion, and spirituality*, edited by Kenneth I. Pargament et al., 713–728. Washington, DC: American Psychological Association, 2013.

Tangney, June P. and Ronda L. Daering. *Shame and guilt.* New York: Guilford Press, 2004.

Taylor, Robert J., Linda M. Chatters and Ann W. Nguyen. "Religious participation and DSM IV major depressive disorder among Black Caribbeans in the United States." *Journal of Immigrant and Minority Health* 15(5) (2013): 903–909.

Tedeschi, Richard G., Crystal L. Park and Lawrence G. Calhoun, eds. *Posttraumatic growth: Positive changes in the aftermath of crisis*. Mahwah, NJ: Erlbaum, 1998.

Tepper, Leslie, Steven A. Rogers, Esther M. Coleman and H. Newton Malony. "The prevalence of religious coping among persons with persistent mental illness." *Psychiatric Services* 52 (2001): 660–665.

Theißen, Gerd. *Urchristliche Wundergeschichten. Ein Beitrag zur formgeschichtlichen Erforschung der synoptischen Evangelien*. Gütersloh: Guetersloher Verlagshaus, 1987.

Thomas, Michael J., Glendon L. Moriarty, Edward B. Davis and Elizabeth L. Anderson. "The Effects of a Manualized Group-Psychotherapy Intervention on Client God Images and Attachment to God: A Pilot Study." *Journal of Psychology and Theology* 39(1) (2011): 44–58.

Thornicroft, Graham, T. Deb and C. Henderson. "Community mental health care worldwide: current status and further developments." *World Psychiatry* 15(3) (2016): 276–286.

Thuné-Boyle, Ingela C., Jan A. Stygall, Mohammed R. Keshtgar and Shanton Newman. "Do religious/spiritual coping strategies affect illness adjustment in patients with cancer? A systematic review of the literature." *Social Science & Medicine* 63 (2006): 151–164.

Toussaint, Loren L., Justin C. Marschall and David R. Williams. "Prospective associations between religiousness/spirituality and depression and mediating effects of forgiveness in a nationally representative sample of United States adults." *Depression Research and Treatment* (2012): 1–10.

Toussaint, Loren L., David R. Williams, Mike A. Musick and Susan A. Everson-Rose. "Why forgiveness may protect against depression: Hopelessness as an explanatory mechanism." *Personality and Mental Health* 2(2) (2008): 89–103.

Troyer, Henry. "Review of cancer among 4 religious sects: Evidence that life-styles are distinctive sets of risk factors." *Social Science & Medicine* 26 (1988): 1007–1017.

Utsch, Michael. *Religiöse Fragen in der Psychotherapie*. Stuttgart: Kohlhammer, 2005.

Utsch, Michael. *Pathologische Religiosität: Genese, Beispiele, Behandlungsansätze*. Stuttgart: Kohlhammer Verlag, 2012.

Utsch, Michael. "Ausschluss oder Einbeziehung spiritueller Interventionen?" In *Psychotherapie und Spiritualität: Mit existenziellen Konflikten und Transzendenzfragen professionell umgehen*, edited by Michael Utsch, Raphael M. Bonelli and Samuel Pfeifer, 111–120. Berlin/Heidelberg: Springer, 2014.

Vail, Kenneth E. et al. "Terror management analysis of the psychological functions of religion." *Personality and Social Psychology Review* 14 (2010): 84–94.

van den Brink, Bart, Hanneke Schaap and Aarjan W. Braam. "Moral Objections and Fear of Hell: An Important Barrier to Suicidality." *Journal of Religion and Health* 57 (2018): 2301–2312.

Vijaykumar, Lakshmi. "Suicide and its prevention: the urgent need in India." *Indian Journal of Psychiatry* 49 (2007): 81–84.

Vittengl, Jeffrey R. "A Lonely Search? Risk for Depression: When Spirituality Exceeds Religiosity." *The Journal of Nervous and Mental Disease* 206 (2018): 386–389.

Von der Heyl, Andreas. *Zwischen Burnout und spiritueller Erneuerung. Studien zum Beruf des evangelischen Pfarrers und der evangelischen Pfarrerin*. Frankfurt am Main: Lang, 2003.

Wachholtz, Amy B. and Elizabeth T. Austin. "Contemporary Spiritual Meditation: Practices and Outcomes." In *APA Handbook of Psychology, Religion, and Spirituality*, edited by Kenneth I. Pargament et al., 311–327. Washington, DC: American Psychological Association, 2013.

Wahass, Saheed and Gerry Kent. "Coping with auditory hallucinations: A cross-cultural comparison between Western (British) and non-Western (Saudi Arabian) patients." *Journal of Nervous and Mental Disease* 185 (1997): 664–668.

Walach, Harald. "Spiritualität als Ressource. Chancen und Probleme eines neuen Forschungsfeldes." *EZW-Texte* 181 (2005): 17–40.

Waller, Heiko. *Gesundheitswissenschaft*, Vol. 2. Stuttgart/Berlin: Kohlhammer, 1996.

WCC (World Council of Churches). *Healing and Wholeness – The Churches Role in Health. The Report of a Study by the Christian Medical Commission*. Geneva: WCC, 1990.

Weber, Friedrich and Michael Strauß. "Burnout–Herausforderung für die Kirche." In *Die auszehrende Organisation*, edited by Dietrich von der Oelsnitz, Frank Schirmer and Kerstin Wüstner, 269–274. Wiesbaden: Springer Gabler, 2014.

Weyel, Birgit. "Christian Communities in the Face of Immigration. Interreligious pastoral care among immigrants." *Salesianum* 81 (2019): 216–232.

Weyel, Birgit and Beate Jakob (eds.). "Spiritualität und Depressivität." In *Menschen mit Depression*, edited by Birgit Weyel et al., 19–26. Gütersloh: Gütersloher Verlagshaus, 2014.

Weyel, Birgit and Beate Jakob (eds.). *Menschen mit Depression: Orientierungen und Impulse für die Praxis in Kirchengemeinden*. Gütersloh: Gütersloher Verlagshaus, 2014.

Weyel, Birgit and Beate Jakob. "Kirchengemeinden als soziales Netz und als Orte der Deutung von Gesundheit / Krankheit." In *Menschen mit Depression*, edited by Birgit Weyel et al., 12–18. Gütersloh: Gütersloher Verlagshaus, 2014.

Wills, Thomas A., Alison M. Yaeger and James M. Sandy. "Buffering effect of religiosity for adolescent substance use." *Psychology of Addictive Behaviors* 17 (2003): 24–31.

Wilson, William P. "Religion and psychoses." In *Handbook of religion and mental health*, edited by Harold G. Koenig, 161–174. New York: Academic Press, 1998.

Wink, Paul, Michaela Dollin and Britta Larsen. "Religion as Moderator of the Depression-Health Connection: Findings from a Longitudinal Study." *Research on Aging* 27(2) (2005): 197–220.

Winkelmann, Judith. "Weil wir nicht vollkommen sein müssen." Zum Umgang mit Belastungen im Pfarrberuf. Stuttgart: Kohlhammer, 2019.

Winkelmann, Judith. "Wie viel von 75% ist unendlich? Strukturelle Faktoren für Burnout als Herausforderung für die Supervision." *Pastoraltheologie* 100(4) (2011): 198–214.

Winkelmann, Sabine. *Religiöse Deutung in schwerer Krankheit.* Berlin/Münster: Lit Verlag, 2016.

Winter, Urs Christian. "*Der Liebe Gott hat es so gewollt*" *: die Rolle der Religiosität bei der Bewältigung kritischer Lebensereignisse sowie Impulse für eine pastorale Krisenintervention – eine pastoralpsychologische Studie* (Dissertation). Fribourg: 2005.

Winter, Urs et al. "The psychological outcome of religious coping with stressful life events in a Swiss sample of church attendees." *Psychotherapy and Psychosomatics* 78 (2009): 240–244.

World Health Organization. *Mental Health Atlas 2017.* Geneva: World Health Organization, 2018.

World Health Organization. "Mental health systems in selected low- and middle-income countries: a WHO-AIMS cross-national analysis," *World Health Organization* (2009): 61.

World Health Organization. *Preamble to the Constitution of WHO as adopted by the International Health Conference.* New York, 19 June – 22 July 1946.

World Health Organization. *Primary Health Care. Report of the International Conference on Primary Health Care, Alma Ata, USSR, 6–12 September.* Geneva: World Health Organization, 1978.

World Health Organization. *Review of the Constitution and Regional Arrangements of the World Health Organization.* EB101/7. Geneva: 1997.

World Health Organization. "The World Health Report 2001: Mental Health: New Understanding, New Hope," *World Health Organization* (2001): 110–112.

Worthington Jr., Everett, Don E. Davis, Joshua N. Hook, Daryl R. van Tongeren, Aubrey L. Gartner, David J. Jennings II, Chelsea L. Greer and Yin Lin. "Religion, Spirituality, and Forgiveness." In *Handbook of the psychology of Religion and Spirituality*, edited by Raymond F. Paloutzian and Crystal L. Park, 476–497. New York: Guilford, 2005.

Wroclawska-Warchala, Emilia and Michal Warchala. "The heavens and hells we believe in. Individual eschatological Images as conditioned by denominational culture." *Archive for the Psychology of Religion* 37 (2015): 240–266.

Yonker, Julie E., Chelsea A. Schnabelrauch and Laura G. DeHaan. "The relationship between spirituality and religiosity on psychological outcomes in adolescents and emerging adults: A meta-analytic review." *Journal of Adolescence* 35 (2012): 299–314.

Young, John L., Ezra E. H. Griffith and David R. Williams. "The integral role of pastoral counseling by African-American clergy in community mental health." *Psychiatric Services* 54(5) (2003): 688–692.

Zinnbauer, Brian J. and Kenneth I. Pargament. "Religiousness and spirituality." In *Handbook of the Psychology of Religion and Spirituality*, edited by Raymond Paloutzian and Crystal L. Park, 21–42. New York: Guilford, 2005.

Znoj, Hansjörg, Christoph Morgenthaler and Christian Zwingmann. “Mehr als nur Bewältigen? Religiosität, Stressreaktionen und Coping bei elterlicher Depressivität nach dem Verlust eines Kindes.“ In *Religiosität: Messverfahren und Studien zu Gesundheit und Lebensqualität. Neue Beiträge zur Religionspsychologie*, edited by Christian Zwingmann and Helfried Moosbrugger, 277–297, Münster: Waxmann, 2004.

Zuckerman, Marvin. *Vulnerability to psychopathology. A biosocial model.* Washington, DC: American Psychological Association, 1999.

Zwingmann, Christian and Bastian Hodapp. “Religiosität/Spiritualität und psychische Gesundheit: Zentrale Ergebnisse einer Metaanalyse über Studien aus dem deutschsprachigen Raum.” *Spiritual Care* 7 (2017): 69–80.

Zwingmann, Christian and Constantin Klein. “Deutschsprachige Fragebogenskalen zur Messung von Religiosität/Spiritualität: Stellenwert, Klassifikation und Auswahlkriterien.” *Spiritual Care* 1(3) (2012): 7–21.

Zwingmann, Christian, Constantin Klein and Florian Jeserich, eds. *Religiosität: Die dunkle Seite: Beiträge zur empirischen Religionsforschung*. Münster/New York: Waxmann, 2017.

Zwingmann, Christian, Constantin Klein and Florian Jeserich. “Ekklesiogene Neurose.” In *Religiosität: Die dunkle Seite: Beiträge zur empirischen Religionsforschung*, edited by Christian Zwingmann, Constantin Klein and Florian Jeserich, 43–64. Münster/New York: Waxmann, 2017.

Zwingmann, Christian, Claudia Müller, Jürgen Körber and Sebastian Murken. “Religious commitment, religious coping and anxiety: A study in German patients with breast cancer.” *European Journal of Cancer Care* 17 (2008): 361–370.

Online Sources

Bündnis gegen Depression. URL: https://www.deutsche-depressionshilfe.de (last accessed on 1 April 2020).

Ebotabe Arrey, Agnes, Johan Bilsen, Patrick Lacor and Reginald Deschepper. "Spirituality/ Religiosity: A Cultural and Psychological Resource among Sub-Saharan African Migrant Women with HIV/AIDS in Belgium." *PLoS ONE* 11(7) (2016). URL: https://doi.org/10.1371/ journal.pone.0159488 (last accessed on 14 May 2019).

Galderisi, Silvana et al. "Toward a new definition of mental health." *World Psychiatry* 14(2) (2015): 231–233. URL: http://doi.org/10.1002/wps.20231 (last accessed on 1 April 2020).

Hefti, René, and Arndt Büssing, eds. *Integrating Religion and Spirituality into Clinical Practice. Conference Proceedings. European Conference on Religion, Spirituality and Health*. URL: https://doi.org/10.3390/books978-3-03842-929-6 (last accessed on 1 April 2020).

Information from WHO. URL: https://www.mhinnovation.net/resources/national-mental-health-strategy-ethiopia (last accessed on 1 April 2020).

Kuttler, Iris. *Pfarrer in der Krise? Zusammenhänge zwischen Arbeitsanforderungen im Pfarrberuf und dem Burnout-Syndrom*. Konstanz 2007. URL: https://d-nb.info/ 1080879579/34 (last accessed on 1 April 2020).

Liste der Länder der Welt nach Lebensaltermedian. URL: https://de.wikipedia.org/wiki/Liste_der_Länder_der_Welt_nach_Lebensaltermedian (last accessed on 1 April 2020).

Malawi International Religious Freedom Report (2014). URL: https://www.state.gov/documents/ organization/238446.pdf (last accessed on 1 April 2020).

Movement for Global Mental Health. URL: http://globalmentalhealth.org/node/190 (last accessed on 1 April 2020).

National Institute of Mental Health. URL: http://www.nimh.nih.gov/health/statistics/global/ global-ylds-contributed-by-mental-and-behavioral-disorders.shtml (last accessed on 1 April 2020).

Rhode, Regina. *Supervision und Ehrenamt – Welche Rahmenbedingungen, Fort- und Weiterbildung brauchen Ehrenamtliche für ihre Arbeit und was kann die Supervision dazu beitragen? Am Beispiel der Ehrenamtlichen Evangelischen Klinikseelsorge der Universitätsklinik Freiburg. Masterthesis, Evangelische Hochschule Freiburg, Masterstudiengang Supervision*. URL: http://arhode.de/regina/files/Masterthesis_ReginaRhode.pdf (last accessed on 1 April 2020).

SEARO – WHO. *Suicide Prevention: Emerging from Darkness* (2001). URL: http://apps.searo.who.int/PDS_DOCS/B0754.pdf (last accessed on 1 April 2020).

Sinha, Suman K. and Jagdish Kaur. "National mental health programme: Manpower development scheme of eleventh five-year plan." *Indian J Psychiatry* 53 (2011): 261–265. URL: https://www.ncbi.nlm.nih.gov/pmc/articles/PMC3221186/ (last accessed on 1 April 2020).

Trevino, Kelly M., Kenneth I. Pargament, Neal Krause, Gail Ironson and Peter Hill. "Stressful Events and Religious/Spiritual Struggle: Moderating Effects of the General Orienting System." *Psychology of Religion and Spirituality* (2017). URL: https://doi.org/10.1037/ rel0000149 (last accessed in December 2018).

IFK Religious Conflicts and Coping Strategies. URL: https://www.religious-conflicts.unibe.ch (last accessed on 1 April 2020).

https://doi.org/10.1515/9783110674217-015

Vigo, Daniel, Graham Thornicroft and Rifat Atun. "Estimating the true global burden of mental illness." *Lancet Psychiatry 3* (2016). URL: https://www.ncbi.nlm.nih.gov/pubmed/26851330 (last accessed on 1 April 2020).

Whiteford, Harvey A. et al. "Global burden of disease attributable to mental and substance use disorders: findings from the Global Burden of Disease Study 2010." URL: www.thelancet.com, published online August 29, 2013: http://dx.doi.org/10.1016/S0140-6736(13)61611-6 (last accessed on 1 April 2020).

World Health Organization. *The Ottawa Charter for Health Promotion. First International Conference on Health Promotion* (Ottawa, 21 November 1986). URL: http://www.who.int/healthpromotion/conferences/previous/ottawa/en/ (last accessed on 20 June 2019).

World Health Organization. "Child and Adolescent Mental Health." URL: http://www.who.int/mental_health/maternal-child/child_adolescent/en/ (last accessed on 1 April 2020).

World Health Organization. "Depression. Fact sheet (January 2020)." URL: https://www.who.int/news-room/fact-sheets/detail/depression (last accessed on 1 April 2020).

World Health Organization. "Fact sheets on mental health (updated March 2018)." URL: https://www.who.int/news-room/fact-sheets/detail/mental-health-strengthening-our-re sponse (last accessed on 1 April 2020).

World Health Organization. "Global Health Observatory data." URL: https://www.who.int/healthinfo/global_burden_disease/en/ (last accessed on 1 April 2020)

World Health Organization. *Mental Health Action Plan 2013 – 2020*. Geneva 2014. URL: http://apps.who.int/iris/bitstream/10665/89966/1/9789241506021_eng.pdf?ua=1 (last accessed on 1 April 2020).

World Health Organization. "Mental health." URL: http://www.who.int/mental_health/en/ (last accessed on 1 April 2020).

World Health Organization. "Mental health: strengthening our response (2018)." URL: http://www.who.int/mediacentre/factsheets/fs220/en/ (last accessed on 1 April 2020).

World Health Organization. "National mental health strategy of Ethiopia." URL: https://www.mhinnovation.net/resources/national-mental-health-strategy-ethiopia (last accessed on 1 April 2020).

World Health Organization & Calouste Gulbenkian Foundation. "Improving access to and appropriate use of medicines for mental disorders (2017)." URL: http://apps.who.int/iris/bitstream/10665/254794/1/9789241511421-eng.pdf?ua=1 (last accessed on 1 April 2020).

Index

https://doi.org/10.1515/9783110674217-016

Printed in the USA
CPSIA information can be obtained
at www.ICGtesting.com
LVHW092012201023
761596LV00004B/423

9 783110 673166